INTERVENTIONAL CARDIOLOGY CLINICS

www.interventional.theclinics.com

Editor-in-Chief

MARVIN H. ENG

Renal Disease Considerations In Coronary, Peripheral and Structural Interventions

October 2023 • Volume 12 • Number 4

Editor

Shweta Bansal

ELSEVIER

1600 John F. Kennedy Boulevard • Suite 1800 • Philadelphia, Pennsylvania, 19103-2899

http://www.theclinics.com

INTERVENTIONAL CARDIOLOGY CLINICS Volume 12, Number 4
October 2023 ISSN 2211-7458, ISBN-13: 978-0-443-12993-3

Editor: Joanna Gascoine
Developmental Editor: Akshay Samson

Interventional Cardiology Clinics (ISSN 2211-7458) is published quarterly by Elsevier Inc., 360 Park Avenue South, New York, NY 10010-1710. Months of issue are January, April, July, and October. Subscription prices are USD 217 per year for US individuals, USD 570 for US institutions, USD 100 per year for US students, USD 217 per year for Canadian individuals, USD 679 for Canadian institutions, USD 100 per year for Canadian students, USD 308 per year for international individuals, USD 679 for international institutions, and USD 150 per year for international students. To receive student/resident rate, orders must be accompanied by name of affiliated institution, date of term, and the *signature* of program/residency coordinator on institution letterhead. Orders will be billed at individual rate until proof of status is received. Foreign air speed delivery is included in all *Clinics* subscription prices. All prices are subject to change without notice. **POSTMASTER:** Send address changes to *Interventional Cardiology Clinics*, Elsevier Health Sciences Division, Subscription Customer Service, 3251 Riverport Lane, Maryland Heights, MO 63043. **Customer Service: Telephone: 1-800-654-2452** (U.S. and Canada); **1-314-447-8871** (outside U.S. and Canada). **Fax: 1-314-447-8029. E-mail: journalscustomerservice-usa@elsevier.com (for print support); journalsonlinesupport-usa@elsevier.com (for online support).**

Reprints. For copies of 100 or more of articles in this publication, please contact the Commercial Reprints Department, Elsevier Inc., 360 Park Avenue South, New York, NY 10010-1710. Tel.: 212-633-3874; Fax: 212-633-3820; E-mail: reprints@elsevier.com.

CONTRIBUTORS

CONSULTING EDITOR

MARVIN H. ENG, MD
Structural Heart Program Medical Director,
Structural Heart Disease Fellowship Director,
Director of Cardiovascular Quality, Banner
University Medical Center, Phoenix, Arizona

EDITOR

SHWETA BANSAL, MBBS, MD, FASN
Professor, Department of Medicine, Division
of Nephrology, UT Health San Antonio,
San Antonio, Texas

AUTHORS

RADHA K. ADUSUMILLI, MD
Nephrology Fellow, The University of Texas
Health Science Center at San Antonio,
San Antonio, Texas

ANUM ASIF, MD
Division of Cardiology, Department of
Medicine, UT Health San Antonio,
San Antonio, Texas

SHWETA BANSAL, MBBS, MD, FASN
Professor, Department of Medicine, Division
of Nephrology, UT Health San Antonio,
San Antonio, Texas

RISHI CHANDIRAMANI, MD
Department of Internal Medicine, Jacobi
Medical Center, Albert Einstein College of
Medicine, Bronx, New York; The Zena and
Michael A. Wiener Cardiovascular Institute,
Icahn School of Medicine at Mount Sinai,
New York, New York

SANJAY CHAUDHARY, MBBS, MD
Department of Critical Care Medicine, Mayo
Clinic, Jacksonville, Florida

STEVEN COCA, DO, MS
Professor of Medicine, Icahn School of
Medicine at Mount Sinai, New York,
New York

EMILY A. EITZMAN
Department of Internal Medicine, Division of
Cardiovascular Medicine, Michigan Medicine,
Ann Arbor, Michigan

AYMAN FATH, MD
Division of Cardiology, Department of
Medicine, UT Health San Antonio,
San Antonio, Texas

PRAKASH S. GUDSOORKAR, MD
Assistant Professor of Medicine, Division of
Nephrology and Kidney Clinical
Advancement, Research and Education CARE
Program, Department of Medicine, University
of Cincinnati, Ohio

HITINDER S. GURM, MBBS
Professor, Internal Medicine, University of
Michigan, Ann Arbor, Michigan

SAMIR R. KAPADIA, MD, FACC, FAHA
Chair, Department of Cardiovascular
Medicine, Heart and Vascular Institute,
Cleveland Clinic, Cleveland, Ohio

KIANOUSH B. KASHANI, MD, MSc, MS
Divisions of Nephrology and Hypertension,
and Pulmonary and Critical Care Medicine,
Department of Medicine, Mayo Clinic,
Rochester, Minnesota

RACHEL G. KROLL, BS
Department of Internal Medicine, Division of
Cardiovascular Medicine, Michigan Medicine,
Ann Arbor, MichiganUSA

YOGAMAYA MANTHA, MD
Division of Cardiology, Department of
Medicine, UT Health San Antonio, San
Antonio, Texas

ROXANA MEHRAN, MD
Center for Interventional Cardiovascular
Research and Clinical Trials, The Zena and
Michael A. Wiener Cardiovascular Institute,
Icahn School of Medicine at Mount Sinai, New
York, New York

ADHYA MEHTA, MD
Department of Internal Medicine, Jacobi
Medical Center, Albert Einstein College of
Medicine, Bronx, New York

JACOB NYSATHER, MD
Nephrology Fellow, Division of Nephrology
and Kidney Clinical Advancement, Research
and Education (CARE) Program, Department
of Medicine, University of Cincinnati, Ohio

ADAM PAMPORI, MD
Clinical Assistant Professor of Medicine,
Department of Cardiovascular Medicine,
Heart and Vascular Institute, Cleveland Clinic,
Cleveland, Ohio

ANAND PRASAD, MD, FACC, FSCAI, RPVI
Division of Cardiology, Department of
Medicine, UT Health San Antonio, San
Antonio, Texas

SHASHANK SHEKHAR, MD
Department of Cardiovascular Medicine,
Heart and Vascular Institute, Cleveland Clinic,
Cleveland, Ohio

RICHARD SOLOMON, MD, FASN, FACP
Emeritus Professor of Medicine, Larner
College of Medicine, University of Vermont,
Burlington, Vermont

ALESSANDRO SPIRITO, MD
The Zena and Michael A. Wiener
Cardiovascular Institute, Icahn School of
Medicine at Mount Sinai, New York,
New York

NADIA R. SUTTON, MD, MPH
Department of Internal Medicine, Division of
Cardiovascular Medicine, Vanderbilt
University Medical Center, Department of
Biomedical Engineering, Vanderbilt University,
Nashville, Tennessee

CHARUHAS V. THAKAR, MD
Department of Medicine, University of
Cincinnati, Professor of Medicine, Division of
Nephrology and Kidney Clinical
Advancement, Research and Education
(CARE) Program, Department of Nephrology,
Veterans Administration Medical Center,
Section Chief, Cincinnati VA Medical Center,
Cincinnati, Ohio

LALITH VEMIREDDY, MD
Nephrology Fellow, Division of
Nephrology, Department of Medicine, UT
Health San Antonio, San Antonio,
Texas

BIRGIT VOGEL, MD
The Zena and Michael A. Wiener
Cardiovascular Institute, Icahn School of
Medicine at Mount Sinai, New York,
New York

PRASANTHI YELAVARTHY, MD
Munson Medical Center, Traverse City,
Michigan

CONTENTS

Foreword   ix
Marvin H. Eng

Preface: Teamwork Makes Success Work   xi
Shweta Bansal

Significance of Kidney Disease in Cardiovascular Disease Patients   453
Adhya Mehta, Rishi Chandiramani, Alessandro Spirito, Birgit Vogel, and
Roxana Mehran

Cardiorenal syndrome is a condition where is a bidirectional and mutually detrimental relationship between the heart and kidneys. The mechanisms underlying cardiorenal syndrome are multifactorial and complex. Patients with
kidney disease exhibit increased cardiovascular risk, presenting as coronary
and peripheral artery disease, structural heart disease, arrhythmias, heart failure, and sudden cardiac death, largely occurring because of a systemic proinflammatory state, causing myocardial and vascular remodeling, manifesting as
atherosclerotic lesions, vascular and valvular calcification, and myocardial fibrosis, particularly among those with advanced disease. This review summarizes
the current understanding and clinical implications of kidney disease in patients
with cardiovascular disease.

Definition, Staging, and Role of Biomarkers in Acute Kidney Injury in the   469
Context of Cardiovascular Interventions
Prakash S. Gudsoorkar, Jacob Nysather, and Charuhas V. Thakar

Acute kidney injury (AKI) is a frequently occurring complication of cardiovascular interventions, and associated with adverse outcomes. Therefore, a clear definition of AKI is of paramount importance to enable timely recognition and
treatment. Historically, changes in the serum creatinine and urine output
have been used to define AKI, and the criteria have evolved over time with better understanding of the impact of AKI on the outcomes. However, the reliance
on serum creatinine for these AKI definitions carries numerous limitations
including delayed rise, inability to differentiate between hemodynamics versus
structural injury and assay variability to name a few.

Contrast-Associated Acute Kidney Injury: Definitions, Epidemiology,   489
Pathophysiology and Implications
Lalith Vemireddy and Shweta Shweta

Acute kidney injury (AKI) is a common occurrence after contrast media administration. Hemodynamic changes, direct tubular injury, and reactive oxygen
species are the proposed mechanisms involved in AKI. However, in most scenarios, it is not possible to establish causality despite extensive clinical evaluation, therefore, contrast-associated AKI (CA-AKI) has become a widely
accepted term to define AKI postcontrast. CA-AKI is associated with worse clinical outcomes including cardiovascular events and mortality; however, discussions are ongoing whether CA-AKI is a marker of an increased risk of
adverse outcomes or a mediator of such outcomes.

Predicting Contrast-induced Renal Complications   **499**
Emily A. Eitzman, Rachel G. Kroll, Prasanthi Yelavarthy, and Nadia R. Sutton

Chronic kidney disease is an independent risk factor for the development of coronary artery disease and overlaps with other risk factors such as hypertension and diabetes. Percutaneous coronary intervention is a cornerstone of therapy for coronary artery disease and requires contrast media, which can lead to renal injury. Identifying patients at risk for contrast-associated acute kidney injury (CA-AKI) is critical for preventing kidney damage, which is associated with both short- and long-term mortality. Determination of the potential risk for CA-AKI and a new need for dialysis using validated risk prediction tools identifies patients at high risk for this complication. Identification of patients at risk for renal injury after contrast exposure is the first critical step in prevention. Contrast media volume, age and sex of the patient, a history of chronic kidney disease and/or diabetes, clinical presentation, and hemodynamic and volume status are factors known to predict incident contrast-induced nephropathy. Recognition of at-risk patient subpopulations allows for targeted, efficient, and cost-effective strategies to reduce the risk of renal complications resulting from contrast media exposure.

Hydration to Prevent Contrast-Associated Acute Kidney Injury in Patients   **515**
Undergoing Cardiac Angiography
Richard Solomon

Administration of fluid (oral and intravenous) is the cornerstone of prevention of contrast-associated acute kidney injury in the cardiac environment. Intravenous saline is the preferred fluid. The amount, timing, and duration of therapy are discussed. A key determinant of the benefit may be the rate of urine output stimulated by the therapy. Approaches using hemodynamic-guided rates of fluid administration and novel techniques to generate large urine outputs while maintaining fluid balance are highlighted.

A Practical Approach to Preventing Contrast-Associated Renal Complications   **525**
in the Catheterization Laboratory
Hitinder S. Gurm

Contrast media use is ubiquitous in the catheterization laboratory. Contrast-associated acute kidney injury (CA-AKI) is a key concern among patients undergoing coronary angiography and percutaneous coronary interventions. The risk of CA-AKI can be minimized by careful attention to hydration status and renal function-based contrast dosing in all patients. In patients with Stage IV chronic kidney disease, ultra low contrast procedure (contrast dose $\leq$ GFR) may be especially beneficial.

Implications of Kidney Disease in Patients with Peripheral Arterial Disease and   **531**
Vascular Calcification
Yogamaya Mantha, Anum Asif, Ayman Fath, and Anand Prasad

Persons with chronic kidney disease (CKD) are at a higher risk of developing peripheral artery disease (PAD) and its adverse health outcomes than individuals with normal renal function. Among patients with CKD, PAD is predominantly characterized by the calcification of the medial layer of arterial vessels in addition to intimal atherosclerosis and calcification. Vascular calcification (VC) is initiated by CKD-associated hyperphosphatemia, hypercalcemia, high concentrations of parathyroid hormone (PTH) as well as inflammation and oxidative stress. VC is widely prevalent in this cohort (>80% dialysis and 50% patients with CKD) and contributes to reduced arterial compliance and symptomatic peripheral arterial disease (PAD). The most severe form of PAD is critical limb ischemia (CLI) which has a substantial risk for increased morbidity and mortality. Percutaneous endovascular interventions with transluminal angioplasty, atherectomy, and intravascular lithotripsy are the current nonsurgical treatments for severe calcific plaque. Unfortunately, there are no randomized controlled trials that address the optimal approach to PAD and CLI revascularization in patients with CKD.

Implications of Renal Disease in Patients Undergoing Structural Interventions   539
Adam Pampori, Shashank Shekhar, and Samir R. Kapadia

Percutaneous structural interventions have a major impact on the morbidity, mortality, and quality of life of patients by providing a lower-risk alternative to cardiac surgery. However, renal disease has a significant impact on outcomes of these interventions. This review explores the incidence, outcomes, pathophysiology, and preventative measures of acute kidney injury and chronic kidney disease on transcatheter aortic valve replacement, transcatheter mitral valve repair, and percutaneous balloon mitral valvuloplasty. Given the expanding indications for percutaneous structural interventions, further research is needed to identify ideal patients with chronic kidney disease or end-stage renal disease who would benefit from intervention.

Acute Kidney Injury Management Strategies Peri-Cardiovascular Interventions   555
Sanjay Chaudhary and Kianoush B. Kashani

In many countries, the aging population and the higher incidence of comorbid conditions have resulted in an ever-growing need for cardiac interventions. Acute kidney injury (AKI) is a common complication of these interventions, associated with higher mortalities, chronic or end-stage kidney disease, readmission rates, and hospital and post-discharge costs. The AKI pathophysiology includes contrast-associated AKI, hemodynamic changes, cardiorenal syndrome, and atheroembolism. Preventive measures include limiting contrast media dose, optimizing hemodynamic conditions, and limiting exposure to other nephrotoxins. This review article outlines the current state-of-art knowledge regarding AKI pathophysiology, risk factors, preventive measures, and management strategies in the peri-interventional period.

Renalism: Avoiding Procedure, More Harm than Good?   573
Radha K. Adusumilli and Steven Coca

Management of patients with chronic kidney disease (CKD) is complex in terms of their disease pathophysiology. Cardiovascular disease is one of the leading causes of death in individuals with CKD. These patients are very prone for developing increase in creatinine usually enough to meet criteria for acute kidney injury spontaneously and after mild insults. The fear of precipitating an acute kidney injury or worsening of CKD (ie, renalism) is preventing current day physicians in providing clinically indicated interventions that have a positive impact on their morbidity and mortality.

RENAL DISEASE CONSIDERATIONS IN CORONARY, PERIPHERAL AND STRUCTURAL INTERVENTIONS

FORTHCOMING ISSUES

January 2024
Multi-Modality Interventional Imaging
Thomas W. Smith, *Editor*

April 2024
Transcatheter Mitral Valves
Firas Zahr and Marvin Eng, *Editors*

July 2024
Interventions for Congenital Heart Disease
Frank Ing and Howaida El-Said, *Editors*

RECENT ISSUES

July 2023
Pulmonary Embolism Interventions
Vikas Aggarwal, *Editor*

April 2023
Intracoronary Imaging and Its Use in
Interventional Cardiology
Yasuhiro Honda, *Editor*

January 2023
Coronary Physiology in Contemporary
Clinical Practice
Allen Jeremias, *Editor*

THE CLINICS ARE NOW AVAILABLE ONLINE!

Access your subscription at:
www.theclinics.com

FOREWORD

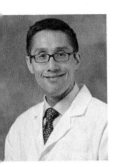

Marvin H. Eng, MD
Consulting Editor

Interventional Cardiology Clinics is pleased to present this issue of Renal Disease Considerations In Coronary, Peripheral And Structural Interventions. Contrast use, cardiogenic shock, and advanced age have significant impact on renal function, which in turn plays a significant role in overall patient survival. Mitigating these risks remains key to the success of any center.

Despite much research, the core of protecting renal function has remained fairly constant. Even so, all interventionalists require an understanding of how to risk-stratify and shield patients from kidney injury. With an overall aging population and more patients with chronic kidney disease, advancing the quality of renal protection stands to benefit nearly everyone. This issue of *Interventional Cardiology Clinics* brings more insight into the pathophysiology of acute kidney injury, contrast-related renal damage, understanding the specifics of different cardiology subgroups, and interventions for preserving renal function.

This issue was edited by Dr Shweta Bansal, a beacon of excellence in nephrology. We congratulate her and her colleagues on a comprehensive and practical issue that will serve anybody caring for cardiology patients.

Marvin H. Eng, MD
Banner University Medical Center
1111 East McDowell Road
Phoenix, AZ 85006, USA

E-mail address:
marvin.eng@bannerhealth.com

https://doi.org/10.1016/j.iccl.2023.08.001
2211-7458/23/© 2023 Published by Elsevier Inc.

PREFACE

Teamwork Makes Success Work

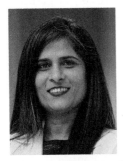

Shweta Bansal, MBBS, MD, FASN
Editor

The prevalence of chronic kidney disease (CKD) has been rising with the epidemic of obesity and its associated comorbidities: diabetes and hypertension. More than 50% of CKD patients have some manifestation of cardiovascular disease (CVD), and CVD rather than end-stage kidney disease is the leading cause of death in this high-risk population. On the other side, increasing numbers of patients with CVD are presenting at a later age with several comorbidities, including CKD, imparting a very high risk for complications, including acute kidney injury (AKI) with any coronary, structural, or peripheral intervention. Patients with CKD are particularly at high risk for AKI after these procedures. Over the last two decades, much has been learned about the short- as well as long-term poor consequences of AKI on an individual's health. That has led many organizations to monitor AKI incidence as a quality metric and take initiatives to reduce these complications.

One of the measures to prevent these periprocedural complications is the act of omission, and the high-risk patients, such as CKD patients, frequently encounter that. Moreover, exclusion of the CKD population from the clinical trials on an intervention does not help the decision making with an unknown risk-benefit ratio. However, absence of evidence does not always conclude a lack of benefit. Recognizing this knowledge gap, many retrospective analyses and a few randomized trials, like TIMI IIIB and TACTICS-TIMI 18,

have included early to moderate CKD patients and demonstrated mortality benefit with early invasive care compared with noninvasive treatment. These analyses inform dire need to include CKD population in these intervention trials to guide the patients and providers. Furthermore, recent interventional trials, like PRESERVE and AMACING, which aimed to reduce the periprocedural complication like AKI, have been shedding light that AKI could be a marker, not the sole mediator, of the poor consequences. It is important to understand that many factors are at play in the patient population requiring cardiovascular intervention, not just the intervention, to cause the complications including AKI. For this issue of *Interventional Cardiology Clinics*, the goal is to update the existing knowledge, present the latest debate, tease association from causality, and discuss the best approach for our patients.

We start by discussing the pathophysiology of cardiorenal interaction to understand why these patients are at high risk for periprocedure complications. Then, we describe the latest methods to define AKI (the most dreaded complication), risk factors for AKI in addition to procedure-related factors, challenges of structural and peripheral interventions, and management strategies to prevent the complications. Finally, we discuss the recent recognition of the fact that these complications could be a marker rather than mediator of the poor consequences postprocedure, and an

Intervent Cardiol Clin 12 (2023) xi–xii
https://doi.org/10.1016/j.iccl.2023.07.001
2211-7458/23/© 2023 Published by Elsevier Inc.

act of omission may not always be the best approach. A multidisciplinary team, including cardiologist, nephrologist, and other providers, executing a thorough assessment of the risk-benefit ratio and discussion with the patient and family to achieve shared decision making are the key to success. I hope you find this issue helpful in contributing to your knowledge and decision making, and enabling the best care to your patients. Meanwhile, I look forward to the new knowledge and research in this area to empower us.

Being asked to serve as the guest editor of this issue has been a great privilege. However, successful production would not have been possible without the expertise, dedication, and time commitment of many individuals. I would like to convey my sincere gratitude to Dr Marvin H. Eng, the editor-in-chief, and Dr Hitinder Gurm, the editor of the previous issue on this topic, to entrust me with this enormous responsibility and their expertise. My deep appreciation to all the authors who generously contributed their time and depth of knowledge to this issue. Last, a huge thanks to the staff of Elsevier, in particular, Mr Akshay Samson and Ms Joanna Collett, for their support, guidance, and cooperation.

Shweta Bansal, MBBS, MD, FASN
Department of Medicine/Division of Nephrology
UT Health San Antonio
7703 Floyd Curl Drive, MSC 7882
San Antonio, TX 78209, USA

E-mail address:
Bansals3@uthscsa.edu

Significance of Kidney Disease in Cardiovascular Disease Patients

Adhya Mehta, MD[a], Rishi Chandiramani, MD[a,b],
Alessandro Spirito, MD[b], Birgit Vogel, MD[b],
Roxana Mehran, MD[c],*

KEYWORDS

- Acute kidney injury • Cardiorenal syndrome • Cardiovascular disease • Chronic kidney disease
- Nephrocardiology

KEY POINTS

- There is a complex bidirectional interaction between cardiac and renal function, with one impacting the other through multiple physiologic pathways.
- This concurrent cardiac and renal dysfunction is broadly termed cardiorenal syndrome and is associated with increased morbidity, increased mortality, and higher economic burden.
- Patients with kidney disease, especially advanced and end stage, exhibit an elevated risk of cardiac events, with cardiovascular causes accounting for almost 50% of deaths in this high-risk population.
- The interplay between cardiac and renal pathologic conditions extends beyond the traditional atherosclerotic risk factors and includes systemic inflammation, oxidative stress, and vascular and valvular calcification.
- With progressive decline in renal function, the burden of both atherosclerotic and nonatherosclerotic pathologic conditions, such as arrhythmia, valvular and arterial calcification, stroke, and sudden cardiac death, increases exponentially, making management even more challenging.

INTRODUCTION

There is a complex interplay between cardiac and renal function, with one impacting the other through multiple physiologic pathways. Interestingly, Robert Bright[1] in 1836 was the first to define the intricate interdependent relationship between the heart and kidneys. This co-dependent relationship where dysfunction of one organ adversely affects the other is broadly termed cardiorenal syndrome (CRS). The shared common pathophysiologic mechanisms responsible for CRS include the hemodynamic interactions between the heart and kidneys in the setting of systemic inflammation, oxidative stress, neurohormonal activation, atherosclerotic disease on both organ systems, alteration of the anemia-inflammation-bone mineral axis in chronic kidney disease (CKD), and structural changes in the heart with eventual heart failure among patients with renal dysfunction.[2] The complex interlink in the pathogenesis of cardiac and renal diseases has amounted to a higher incidence of cardiac disease in patients with renal illnesses and vice versa. Consequently,

[a] Department of Internal Medicine, Jacobi Medical Center/Albert Einstein College of Medicine, 1400 Pelham Parkway South, Bronx, NY 10461, USA; [b] The Zena and Michael A. Wiener Cardiovascular Institute, Icahn School of Medicine at Mount Sinai, One Gustave L. Levy Place, Box 1030, New York, NY 10029, USA; [c] Center for Interventional Cardiovascular Research and Clinical Trials, The Zena and Michael A. Wiener Cardiovascular Institute, Icahn School of Medicine at Mount Sinai, One Gustave L. Levy Place, Box 1030, New York, NY 10029-6574, USA
* Corresponding author.
E-mail address: roxana.mehran@mountsinai.org

Intervent Cardiol Clin 12 (2023) 453–467
https://doi.org/10.1016/j.iccl.2023.06.006

the coexistence of cardiac and renal dysfunction is associated with increased mortality, increased morbidity, and higher economic burden.[3,4] Therefore, this review aims to describe the prevalence of kidney disease (both acute and chronic) in patients with cardiovascular disease (CVD), provide an overview of the complex cardiorenal interactions, and elaborate on the various management strategies for CRS.

EPIDEMIOLOGY

The global prevalence of CKD and CVD in 2017 was estimated to be 697.5 million and 485.6 million, respectively.[5,6] Notably, around half of the patients with advanced CKD have associated CVD.[7] Furthermore, renal impairment in the form of CKD or worsening renal failure has been attributed as one of the strongest predictors of poor outcomes in patients with heart disease, being independently associated with new cardiovascular events, increased incidence of rehospitalization as well as short- and long-term mortality in patients with chronic coronary artery disease (CAD) and congestive heart failure (CHF).[8,9] A meta-analysis including 1.3 million subjects reported an exponential increase in all-cause mortality with worsening renal function, with cardiovascular deaths constituting the majority.[10] In fact, CVD has been reported to account for nearly 40% to 50% of deaths in patients with advanced (stage 4) or end-stage dialysis-dependent (stage 5) CKD compared with 26% in those with normal kidney function.[11,12]

DEFINITION

As per the Consensus Conference by the Acute Dialysis Quality Group, CRS is an umbrella term used to identify a disorder of the heart and kidneys, whereby acute or chronic dysfunction in one organ may induce acute or chronic dysfunction in the other organ.[13] As per the classification proposed, it is broadly divided into 2 main groups: cardiorenal and renocardiac syndromes, depending on the primary pathologic condition, and further into five subtypes based on the chronicity (Table 1).[13] These are as follows.

- *Acute CRS (type I):* Acute cardiac function deterioration leading to renal injury and/or dysfunction.
- *Chronic CRS (type II):* Chronic abnormalities in cardiac function leading to renal injury and/or dysfunction.
- *Acute renocardiac syndrome (type III):* Worsening acute kidney function/acute kidney injury (AKI) leading to heart injury and/or dysfunction.
- *Chronic renocardiac syndrome (type IV):* CKD leading to heart injury, disease, and/or dysfunction.
- *Secondary CRS (type V):* Simultaneous injury and/or dysfunction of the heart and kidney.[13] This subtype is caused by a systemic illness that causes simultaneous dysfunction of the heart and kidney and lacks a primary organ dysfunction (Table 2).

Table 1
Classification of cardiorenal syndrome

Type	Primary Pathologic Condition	Cause of Morbidity
Type 1 (acute cardiorenal)	Acute cardiac dysfunction leading to AKI	Multiple acute causes (ACS, arrhythmias, valvular heart disease, venous congestion, and so forth) causing ADHF/cardiogenic shock and resulting in AKI
Type 2 (chronic cardiorenal)	Chronic cardiac dysfunction leading to renal dysfunction	Chronic heart failure
Type 3 (acute renocardiac)	AKI leading to cardiac dysfunction	Heart failure in the setting of AKI from volume overload, systemic inflammation, and metabolic abnormalities
Type 4 (chronic renocardiac)	CKD leading to cardiac dysfunction	Myocardial remodeling and dysfunction from CKD-associated cardiomyopathy
Type 5 (secondary cardiorenal)	Systemic condition leading to both cardiac and renal dysfunction	Endocrinologic, autoimmune, sepsis, drugs

Table 2 Causes of cardiorenal syndrome type V	
Acute Causes	**Chronic Causes**
Sepsis	Diabetes mellitus
Infections (malaria, leptospira, parvovirus B19, cytomegalovirus, coxsackie virus, toxoplasmosis)	Hypertension
Drugs/toxins (chemotherapy, cocaine, heroin, CCB, arsenic, snake bite, scorpion bite)	Amyloidosis
Vasculitis/thrombotic microangiopathy	Autoimmune (SLE, sarcoidosis)
Endocrinologic (pheochromocytoma)	Chronic liver disease

Abbreviations: CCB, calcium channel blockers; SLE, systemic lupus erythematosus.

It is important to note that various pathophysiologic mechanisms play a role in driving CRS, and that one type of CRS can progress into another. A retrospective study of 30,681 patients, who had at least one echocardiography at a single health system, demonstrated that 8% of all study participants developed at least one of the subtypes of CRS. Most patients developed an acute form of CRS (type I and III), and up to 19% of patients with chronic CRS subsequently developed an acute syndrome. Development of acute or type IV CRS is independently associated with mortality (myocardial infarction [MI] and stroke), with the acute form carrying the worst prognosis. [14]

PATHOPHYSIOLOGY OF CARDIORENAL INTERACTIONS

Traditional Risk Factors of Vascular Disease in Kidney Disease

Traditional cardiovascular risk factors, such as hypertension, diabetes mellitus, dyslipidemia, and smoking, are widely prevalent in patients with kidney disease.[15] Their role in the progression of both atherosclerotic cardiovascular disease (ASCVD) and CKD is particularly important because of their effect on microvasculature as well as larger vessels.[16,17]

Although elevated cardiovascular risk among patients with CKD cannot be solely explained by elevated blood pressure (BP), treatment of hypertension is known to be beneficial in these patients, as also supported by the results of the SPRINT (Systolic Blood Pressure Intervention Trial) trial.[18] Neurohormonal mechanisms are activated in heart failure as a result of impaired baroreceptor reflex and result in overactivity of sympathetic nervous system and the renin-angiotensin-aldosterone system (RAAS) (Fig. 1).[19] Angiotensin II (AT) has been widely known to cause pressure-induced renal injury via its ability to induce glomerular and systemic hypertension resulting in proteinuria.[20] Moreover, an increase in AT levels can be detrimental to the heart by causing cell death via vasoconstriction and myocardial tissue necrosis through various physiologic mechanisms.[21,22] The sodium and fluid retention along with systemic vasoconstriction via the RAAS pathway worsens systemic

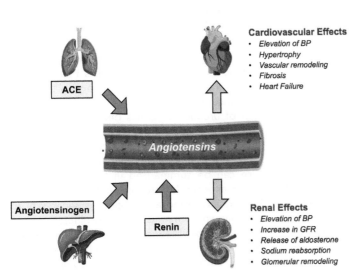

Fig. 1. Role of the RAAS in CRS. GFR, glomerular filtration rate.

Cardiovascular Effects
- *Elevation of BP*
- *Hypertrophy*
- *Vascular remodeling*
- *Fibrosis*
- *Heart Failure*

Renal Effects
- *Elevation of BP*
- *Increase in GFR*
- *Release of aldosterone*
- *Sodium reabsorption*
- *Glomerular remodeling*

ACE

Angiotensins

Angiotensinogen

Renin

congestion and adds to the stress of the heart. AT-1 receptors upregulation and raised AT levels further contribute to cardiac remodeling.[23–26] In addition, AT also contributes to the production of reactive oxygen species and systemic inflammation via receptors AT-1 and AT-2.[21]

Improved glycemic control in patients with type 2 diabetes mellitus has been found to reduce microvascular complications, such as nephropathy and retinopathy, with inconsistent effects on macrovascular events. Among more than 11,000 patients included in the ADVANCE (Action in Diabetes and Vascular Disease: Preterax and Diamicron Modified Release Controlled Evaluation) trial, intensive glucose control (hemoglobin A_{1c} <7%) led to a reduction in the combined outcome of major macrovascular and microvascular events primarily driven by a reduction in nephropathy.[27]

With regard to lipid profile, it has been found that progressive renal dysfunction may drastically change the composition and distribution of blood lipids, particularly high-density lipoprotein (HDL) and triglycerides, to create a more atherogenic environment.[28] Notably, the adverse endothelial effects of HDL have been reported among children with CKD in whom other inflammatory conditions, diabetes, hypertension, or active infections were not yet present.[29] Factors associated with this modification of the HDL molecule in patients with CKD include accumulation of uremic toxins, such as symmetric dimethylarginine, increased oxidative stress, and a proinflammatory milieu.[28]

Nontraditional Risk Factors of Vascular Disease in Kidney Disease
Inflammation
Both CKD and CVD are states of heightened chronic inflammation as a result of abnormalities of neurohormones, particularly elevated RAAS, venous congestion, and ischemia. Inflammatory cytokines, such as interleukin-1 beta (IL-1β), IL-4, IL-6, and tumor necrosis factor (TNF)-α, are known to facilitate accelerated atherosclerosis, cardiac hypertrophy, dysfunction, and fibrosis.[30] IL-1β, in particular, is fundamental in maintenance of cardiac dysfunction in CRS type 3. Simultaneously, activation of the nuclear factor kappa B signaling pathway owing to an increase in renal expression of IL-6 and TNF-α causes a decline in renal function (Fig. 2).[31] Consistent with this, a subanalysis of the CANTOS (Canakinumab Anti-Inflammatory Thrombosis Outcomes Study), which involved more than 10,000 stable post-MI patients with persistently elevated high-sensitivity C-reactive protein, found that IL-1β inhibition with canakinumab reduced major adverse cardiovascular event rates in the CKD population as well.[32]

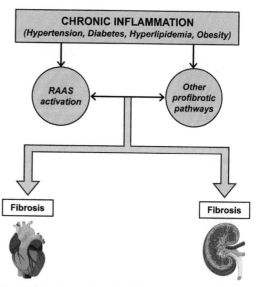

Fig. 2. Cardiac and renal dysfunction among patients with chronic inflammation in the setting of systemic illness.

In recent years, more has been learned about the role of damage-associated molecular patterns (DAMPs) in promoting inflammation and propagate CRS. DAMPs are endogenous molecules that are released from damaged cells, such as after ischemia or under stress, with a purpose to activate the innate immune system and proliferative phase to repair the damage. Although DAMPs are released to contribute to the host's defense, these may promote pathologic inflammatory responses. DAMPs activate inflammation by either of the 2 signal pathways, the NLRP3 signaling pathway or the classical toll-like receptor (TLR2/4) pathway, through TLRs on multiple cells, such as cardiomyocytes, cardiac macrophages, fibroblasts, and inflammatory cells, which release IL-1β in response.[33,34]

Uremic toxins and metabolic derangements
Uremic toxins refer to molecules that accumulate in the bloodstream secondary to impaired clearance owing to renal dysfunction. Accumulation of uremic toxins has been observed in all types of CRS, specifically types 3 and 4, whereby the primary injury is to the kidney. The adverse effects of uremia and uremic toxins on vasculature can be summarized in the four following major aspects: (a) promotion of plaque formation by increasing atherosclerosis secondary to vascular smooth muscle cell proliferation and plaque destabilization by increasing prothrombotic factors, such as von Willebrand factor and thrombomodulin; (b) loss of compliance of

vascular wall causing arterial stiffness; (c) increase in vascular calcification mainly owing to inorganic phosphate, cytokines, and oxidative stress; (d) abnormalities in vascular repair and neointimal hyperplasia owing to vascular smooth muscle cell proliferation, decrease in endothelial progenitor cells, and impairment of wound repair mechanisms by uremia and protein bounds uremic toxins.[35]

Uric acid, frequently elevated in renal dysfunction, is associated with negative cardiovascular effects, such as endothelial dysfunction, increased RAAS activity, inflammation, oxidative stress, and functional abnormalities (Fig. 3). It promotes vascular, cardiac, and renal fibrosis as well.[36] Various nondialyzable protein-bound uremic toxins, indoxyl sulfate, and p-cresol sulfate have been associated with progression of CKD, increased oxidative stress on the heart, and cardiac fibrosis.[37,38]

The other significant abnormalities present in CKD is hyperphosphatemia owing to reduced renal clearance and decreased 1,25 (OH)$_2$ vitamin D levels, that leads to secondary hyperparathyroidism. Elevated inorganic phosphorous and parathyroid hormone (PTH) in CKD correlate with the progression of cardiac and renal dysfunction. These are associated with ventricular hypertrophy, vascular and visceral calcification, CVD, and mortality.[39,40] Over the last decade, klotho–Fibroblast growth factor-23 (FGF23) axis has earned much attention as the mediator of cardiorenal connections. Klotho expression is reduced as soon as kidney function starts deteriorating, generating a state of FGF23 resistance. FGF23 levels also increase early in CKD in response to inflammation and later owing to phosphate retention. The activation of Wnt/β-catenin signaling pathways has been attributed as a cause as well as a consequence of klotho reduction and FGF23 elevation in CKD. Eventually, the Wnt/β-catenin activation mediates the injury in both heart and kidney through the renin-angiotensin system, atherosclerosis, vascular calcification, endothelial dysfunction, cardiac fibrosis, and hypertrophy.[41,42]

Epigenetics

There is evidence to suggest a role of epigenetic modifications in all five types of CRS. However,

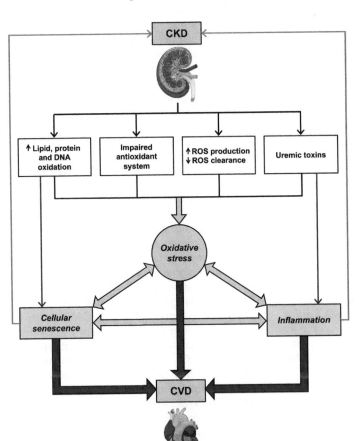

Fig. 3. Interplay between renal and cardiovascular systems in the presence of oxidative stress. ROS, reactive oxygen species.

the direct effects of histone modification, gene methylation, phosphorylation, and micro-RNA (miRNA) on CRS are not known. Histone modification leads to activation of cardiomyopathy-related genes. Histones also undergo modification during renal cell injury.[43] Micro-RNA 21 (miR-21) is the common miRNA that has been studied for its involvement in the pathogenesis of CRS and is found to be expressed in all 5 types of CRS. MiR-21 is activated by inflammation, apoptosis, and fibrosis. It is reported to be overexpressed in the heart and kidneys after injury, causing acute worsening of primary organ dysfunction in CRS and progression from acute to chronic dysfunction.[44] In the heart, miR-21 activates fibroblasts and growth hormone secretion, leading to fibrosis and remodeling after injury.[45]

Vascular and valvular calcification
Vascular smooth muscle cells in the tunica media of blood vessels switch to osteoblastic-like cells in response to CKD-associated bone-mineral abnormalities, inflammation, and oxidative stress.[46] As aforementioned, CKD is associated with hyperphosphatemia and elevated PTH, which regulates calcium and phosphorus levels. However, prolonged elevation of PTH levels in CKD can lead to increased release of calcium and phosphate from the bones into the bloodstream. In addition, CKD is also associated with reduced calcification inhibitors like pyrophosphate, matrix Gla protein, and fetuin.[47] Overall, these abnormalities and uremic milieu promote vascular and valvular calcification.[48,49] Interestingly, coronary artery calcification has been commonly identified even among young adults with end-stage renal disease (ESRD) who are undergoing dialysis.[50] This vascular calcification plays an important role in increased pulse wave velocity, earlier reflection of the pulse wave, and increased afterload, which can lead to left ventricular hypertrophy (LVH) and ultimately to heart failure.[51,52] Within the heart, the aortic and mitral valves are particularly susceptible to calcification.[53] This condition is commonly observed in patients with advanced CKD, particularly those on dialysis, although it can occur at any stage of kidney disease.[53] Over time, these structural changes in the valves cause valvular stenosis or regurgitation.[48,53]

Left Ventricular Hypertrophy in Kidney Disease
In CKD, LVH develops because of multiple interconnected mechanisms, as described above. Afterload-related factors, such as increased arterial stiffness, resulting in increased systemic arterial resistance, and hypertension certainly play an important part.[54] Another major driving force is volume overload and systemic congestion, which leads to length extension of myocardial cells, and eccentric left ventricular remodeling.[54] Concurrently, neurohormonal activation, interference with the normal cellular signaling pathways in the myocardium by uremic toxins, inflammation, myocardial fibrosis, calcium-handling abnormalities, anemia-induced tissue hypoxia, and genetic factors all play a role in development of LVH among patients with CKD.[54]

MANAGEMENT STRATEGIES
Diagnosis of Vascular Disease in Patients with Chronic Kidney Disease
Diagnosis of CAD in patients with renal dysfunction remains challenging. There are limited data on this high-risk population, as patients with CKD are underrepresented in clinical trials.[55] Hence, it is difficult to extrapolate study findings to patients with advanced CKD. Moreover, in addition to higher burden of atherosclerosis, progressive decline in renal function associates with high burden of nonatherosclerotic pathologic conditions, such as arrhythmia, valvular and arterial calcification, stroke, and sudden cardiac death (SCD), exceeding the proportional increase in atherosclerotic pathologic conditions, making management even more challenging.[56]

The choice of diagnostic procedures is limited in these patients because of either decreased renal clearance of pharmacologic agents used or variable efficacy of tests in this population. Functional testing, such exercise stress test or pharmacologic perfusion imaging, have reduced accuracy for detecting CAD in CKD.[57] A meta-analysis concluded that the sensitivity of dobutamine stress echocardiogram and myocardial perfusion scintigraphy was moderate in detecting coronary artery stenosis among patients undergoing transplantation.[57] Stress testing is also limited by a higher proportion of existing baseline electrocardiographic abnormalities (LVH, ST-T wave changes) in these patients.[58] Therefore, coronary artery calcium (CAC) score or computed tomography angiography (CTA) may be more beneficial than functional testing in patients with CKD.[59] In fact, CTA demonstrated higher sensitivity (93%) than CAC score (67%) or single-photon emission computerized tomography (SPECT) (53%) in detecting coronary artery stenosis of greater than 50%.[59] However, one must be mindful of the risk of contrast-associated AKI (CA-AKI) with CTA and the utility of noninvasive tests, such as SPECT, in this situation.[60] Finally, commonly used biomarkers of cardiac injury, such as troponins, can be elevated in patients with CKD without acute coronary syndrome (ACS). This low level of elevation likely occurs owing to myocardial stunning during dialysis or cardiac hypertrophy in patients with CKD.[61,62] Thus, it is essential to use a combination of diagnostics to evaluate cardiac dysfunction in patients with CKD.

Treatment of Vascular Disease in Patients with Chronic Kidney Disease

Controlling traditional cardiovascular risk factors, such as diabetes and hypertension, helps prevent progression of CAD and renal failure. The target BP in patients with CKD has been a topic of continued debate. Although the most recent update of KDIGO in 2021 supports a systolic BP goal of less than 120 mm Hg when tolerated, the European Society of Cardiology guidelines of 2021 recommend a systolic BP target of 130 to 139 mm Hg and a diastolic BP target of less than 80 mm Hg.[63,64] Thus, the generalized consensus is to tailor BP based on individual patient factors, such as tolerability, comorbidities, and proteinuria.[65] Patients with diabetes are at elevated risk of macrovascular (cardiovascular) and microvascular (retinopathy, nephropathy) complications. A reduction and strict control of hemoglobin A_{1c} has been associated with reduction of microvascular complications but no clear benefit in cardiovascular complications.[66–68] In fact, the ACCORD (Action to Control Cardiovascular Risk in Diabetes) trial reported an increase in cardiovascular mortality and an increase in hypoglycemic events with intensive A_{1c} control (<6%).[66,69] Therefore, blood glucose targets must be individualized to avoid hypoglycemic events, especially in patients with CKD because of impaired insulin clearance. Sodium-glucose cotransporter-2 (SGLT2) inhibitors, a class of antidiabetic drugs, have been found to reduce incidence of cardiovascular mortality and prevent the progression of renal dysfunction in addition to control of blood sugar.[70] In addition, glucagon-like peptide-1 agonists have also been associated with a reduction in ASCVD outcomes, such as cardiovascular mortality, nonfatal MI in patients with diabetes, and CVD.[71–73]

The evidence supporting a reduction in cardiovascular events/mortality by lipid-lowering therapies, such as statins, is mixed. These therapies have demonstrated relative reduction in cardiovascular mortality, nonfatal MI, nonfatal stroke, or coronary revascularization among patients with CKD; however, no such benefit has been reported among dialysis-dependent patients with CKD.[74–76] Using protein convertase subtilisin/kexin type 9 (PCSK9) inhibitors with statins in patients with CKD has been reported to be more beneficial than statins alone. Although a study reported that reduction in cardiovascular events with evolocumab, a PCSK9 inhibitor, extended across various stages of CKD, patients with an estimated glomerular filtration rate (eGFR) < 20 mL/min/m^2 and renal transplant were excluded from the study population.[77]

The optimal strategy and duration of antiplatelet therapy for primary and secondary prevention of cardiovascular events in patients with CKD is an important area of research.[78–80] This is because CKD as a risk factor is associated not only with increased thrombotic risk but also with high bleeding risk.[81] Moreover, patients with CKD are highly underrepresented in trials evaluating invasive therapies (percutaneous coronary intervention or coronary artery bypass graft) versus medical therapy among patients with established CAD, which makes determining an optimal strategy for this high-risk population even more complicated.[81] A meta-analysis of patients with CKD admitted for unstable angina or non-ST segment elevation MI reported no significant reduction in all-cause mortality or nonfatal MI but lower rates of rehospitalization in those undergoing invasive management for ACS.[82] The International Study of Comparative Health Effectiveness with Medical and Invasive Approaches–Chronic Kidney Disease (ISCHEMIA-CKD) trial compared an invasive or conservative approach in patients with stable CAD but with positive moderate to severe ischemia on stress test and CKD. No difference in the primary composite end point of death or nonfatal MI was reported between the 2 groups; however, the invasive strategy arm was associated with higher rates of death or initiation of dialysis as well as stroke compared with the conservative strategy arm.[83]

Despite major advancements in the field of cardiology allowing for increasing number of minimally invasive diagnostic and interventional procedures, CA-AKI remains a dreaded complication in patients receiving intravascular radiocontrast media.[84] The definition, risk factors, pathophysiology, prediction, and prevention strategies of CA-AKI are discussed in the other sections of this issue.

Treatment of Patients with Heart Failure and Chronic Kidney Disease

Management of renal or cardiac dysfunction in CRS is mostly focused on diagnosing and treating the primary pathologic condition. Because venous congestion is one of the major mechanisms of CRS, vascular decongestion becomes the most important part of treatment. Diuretics are used to decrease the circulating blood volume, especially in patients with type 1 and 2 CRS. However, because of altered hemodynamics, the volume of distribution and diuretics being protein-bound, patients with CKD might require a higher dose of diuretics for the same effect. Importantly, one must be mindful of electrolyte disturbances, disruption of the neurohormonal balance, and worsening of renal function owing to rapid diuresis or overdiuresis.[2,19] Overall, the role of diuretics in providing a mortality benefit in CRS is not well established.

Beta-blockers and RAAS inhibitors constitute the first-line drugs for management of heart failure with reduced ejection fraction (HFrEF). A subanalysis of the MERIT-HF (Metoprolol CR/XL Randomised Intervention Trial in Congestive Heart Failure) trial showed similar efficacy of long-acting metoprolol in reducing death and hospitalizations for worsening heart failure between patients with decreased renal function (eGFR <45 mL/min/1.73 m^2) and those with eGFR greater than 60 mL/min/1.73 m^2.[85] Another meta-analysis also concluded that treatment with beta-blockers led to an improvement in all-cause mortality in patients with CKD.[86] Nonetheless, beta-blockers were associated with increased risk of bradycardia and hypotension.[86] Hence, they need to be used judiciously, especially among patients with acute CRS.

Different components of the RAAS axis have been targeted by agents such as angiotensin-converting enzyme (ACE) inhibitors, angiotensin receptor blockers (ARB), angiotensin receptor/neprilysin inhibitor, and direct renin inhibitors. ACE inhibitors have proven to be beneficial in patients with CHF and renal dysfunction in outpatient settings.[87,88] The SOLVD (Studies of Left Ventricular Dysfunction) trial showed reduced mortality and hospitalization with the addition of enalapril to conventional therapy among patients with HFrEF (left ventricular ejection fraction < 35%, serum creatinine < 2 mg/dL).[89] The enalapril group reported a higher risk of an increase in serum creatinine; however, no data were provided on the progression of CKD.[89] Nonetheless, a post hoc analysis reported beneficial effects of enalapril with reduced risk for all-cause mortality, even at moderate and severely depressed levels of baseline eGFR.[90] Moreover, it did not seem to harm kidney function.[90] A study comprising 1665 patients receiving ACE inhibitors or ARBs deduced that prescription of these medications was associated with a reduction in all-cause mortality in older patients with systolic heart failure and CKD, including those with more advanced CKD.[91] However, it is important to note that hyperkalemia is a common side effect, especially in patients with renal dysfunction.

As aldosterone can cause fibrosis and myocardial injury, direct blockade of action by mineralocorticoid receptor antagonist (MRA) is important.[88–90] Spironolactone and eplerenone have been shown to improve the prognosis of patients with HFrEF and CKD stages 1 to 3.[91] Finerenone, a novel nonsteroidal selective MRA, also showed a lower risk of progression of CKD and cardiovascular events in patients with CKD and type 2 diabetes mellitus.[92] However, no significant benefit in diastolic dysfunction and cardiac function in patients with advanced CKD has been reported. Moreover, an increased frequency of moderate hyperkalemia was reported.[93,94] Therefore, given the lack of strong evidence supporting the use and the adverse effects, this class of medications has not gained the status of standard of care in patients with advanced CKD.

Although inotropes such as dobutamine, dopamine, and milrinone are used to treat patients with low BP to maintain adequate organ perfusion, they do not necessarily improve outcomes. The OPTIME-CHF (Outcomes of a Prospective Trial of Intravenous Milrinone for Exacerbations of a Chronic Heart Failure) trial reported that use of milrinone in patients with acute decompensated heart failure (ADHF) did not improve kidney function or overall survival.[95] Contrarily, the DAD-HF (Dopamine in Acute Decompensated Heart Failure) trial found the combination of low-dose furosemide with low-dose dopamine was equally effective as high-dose furosemide and associated with improved renal function and potassium homeostasis.[96] Thus, inotropes along with diuretics can be a helpful strategy for the management of appropriate patients with CRS types 1 or 2.

Sodium nitroprusside helps reduce vascular congestion by increasing venous and/or arterial dilation and decreasing myocardial oxygen consumption. Furthermore, it has been associated with hemodynamic improvements and decreased all-cause mortality, irrespective of inotropic support or renal dysfunction.[97] However, one must be mindful of accumulation of thiocyanate in patients with renal dysfunction.[98] Adenosine antagonists can increase urine output by selectively blocking adenosine A1 receptors and allowing the binding of A2 receptors. Nevertheless, a trial evaluating rolofylline, an adenosine A1 receptor antagonist, in patients with ADHF with renal dysfunction did not find any significant improvement in renal function or 60-day outcomes. Furthermore, the overall adverse effect rates between groups were similar; however, only patients in the rolofylline group had seizures.[99] Notably, SGLT2 inhibitors have shown immense benefit in patients with heart failure and renal dysfunction regardless of their diabetes status. They have been found to improve cardiovascular mortality and decrease the progression of renal failure.[100–102]

Eventually, renal replacement therapy/ultrafiltration (UF) via dialysis for removal of excess fluid and uremic toxins might be needed in patients with volume overload, diuretic resistance, hyperkalemia, advanced CKD, and uremic symptoms. The UNLOAD (Ultrafiltration versus Intravenous Diuretics for Patients Hospitalized for Acute Decompensated Heart Failure) trial of patients with ADHF showed that UF produced greater weight and fluid loss than intravenous diuretics, while also reducing 90-day resource utilization for heart failure.[103] However, the Cardiorenal Rescue Study in Acute Decompensated Heart Failure (CARRESS) trial, which focused on patients with CRS, found that use of stepped pharmacologic therapy was superior to UF for the preservation of renal function at 96 hours, with similar amount of weight loss in both arms.[104] In fact, higher rates of complications were noted in the UF arm.[104] Furthermore, the AVOID-HF (Aquapheresis Versus Intravenous Diuretics and Hospitalizations for Heart Failure) trial found that while patients undergoing adjustable UF trended toward a longer time to first heart failure event, they were also more likely to experience a special interest or serious product-related adverse event.[105] Hence, the decision for invasive removal of fluid needs to be taken on a case-by-case basis.

Prevention of Arrhythmias and Sudden Cardiac Death in Chronic Kidney Disease

There is a high incidence of SCD in patients with CKD; however, the exact incidence is unknown.[106] Dialysis is a strong risk factor for SCD, likely because of the sudden volume shifts and electrolyte changes associated with it.[107] Other mechanisms include long-term changes in myocardium and vasculature, uremia, and volume overload. Antiarrhythmic agents and implantable cardioverter-defibrillators (ICDs) have proven beneficial in the general population; however, their use in patients with CKD remains controversial. A meta-analysis reported increased mortality in patients with CKD who received ICD.[108] Although ventricular fibrillation is the most common rhythm in SCD, there have been increased reports of bradyarrhythmia preceding asystole in patients with CKD, which might be a cause of decreased benefit of ICD implantation in this population.[109,110]

Treatment of Valvular Disease in Chronic Kidney Disease

Aortic and mitral valves are most commonly affected in patients with CKD. As there is a lack of isolated guidelines for management of valvular diseases in patients with CKD, decisions for intervention are extrapolated from the guidelines for the general population. Medical therapy can neither reverse nor halt the progression of valvular dysfunction in patients with CKD, making intervention essential.[111] Advanced CKD (eGFR <20 mL/min/m^2) is an independent predictor of mortality and perioperative/permanent dialysis after valvular surgery.[112] Therefore, renal function is included as an important parameter of the scoring system to calculate the preoperative risk and guide the choice of procedure.[113]

In the general population, transcatheter aortic valve replacement (TAVR) has shown superiority over surgical aortic valve replacement in mortality and stroke outcomes.[114,115] Notably, a study with patients with advanced CKD reported better outcomes with transcatheter approach compared with surgical approach as well.[116] However, preexisting CKD (eGFR <60 mL/min/m^2) was reported as a strong predictor of worse short- and long-term outcomes following TAVR. This vulnerable study population had worse 30-day mortality, cardiovascular mortality, strokes, AKI, and the risk for dialysis.[111]

Mitral valvular pathologic conditions treated by surgical repair have better outcomes compared with surgical reconstruction.[113] However, patients with CKD have worse mortality outcomes even with surgical repair. The risk of mortality worsens with deterioration of renal function, increasing from 13% in early stages of CKD to 33% in advanced stages and ESRD.[117] Because there remains a paucity of data on this subject, decisions regarding need for intervention and the type of repair in patients with CKD would require a multidisciplinary approach involving cardiology, nephrology, and primary care.

Potential Therapeutic Targets

FGF23 is a potential target for preventing progression of CRS and its adverse effects on organs. Direct inhibition of action by FGF23 neutralizing antibodies and FGF23 receptor blockade have both been tried. Neutralization of FGF23 was found to cause a sustained decrease in PTH levels and improvement of calcium–vitamin D homeostasis.[118] However, a dose-dependent increase in serum phosphate and aortic calcification associated with an increased risk of mortality was observed in the rat model, which limited its use.[118] FGF23 receptor blockade attenuated LVH in animal models and is a potential therapeutic strategy.[41] In the same animal model, it was observed that besides klotho-related mechanisms, FGF23 also produced its adverse effects via other pathways. Therefore, isolated klotho repletion would not be effective.[41] Moreover, it is important to note that vitamin D supplementation and dietary phosphorous restriction can also decrease the serum level of FGF23 and its cardiotoxic adverse effects.[119] In addition, vitamin D attenuates LVH, decreases FGF4 receptor expression, and suppresses PTH.[37,119]

Other interesting potential therapeutic targets studied in animal models include the TLR signaling pathways, which involve inflammasomes that play a major role in sustaining cardiac myocyte dysfunction, and silencing of miRNA that have proven to be effective in attenuating the progression of cardiac fibrosis and organ dysfunction.[45,120,121] However, these strategies still need to be explored further with more evidence.

SUMMARY

A complex interaction occurs between the heart and kidneys via various hemodynamic, neurohormonal, and metabolic pathways. In addition to traditional risk factors, such as hypertension, diabetes mellitus, dyslipidemia, and smoking, nontraditional risk factors, such as inflammation, uremic toxins, and vascular/valvular calcification, also play an important role in the pathophysiology of CRS. It is pertinent for clinicians to understand the nuances and bidirectional impact of these interactions in order to manage both cardiovascular and renal conditions appropriately. Approaching the management of vascular disease, valvular disorders, arrhythmias, and eventual heart failure holistically, keeping in mind the higher risk and limitations with regard to diagnostic and therapeutic modalities, in patients with dysfunction involving both organ systems simultaneously, is key to improving patient outcomes.

CLINICS CARE POINTS

- Cardiac dysfunction and renal dysfunction are closely interrelated and often exacerbate one another. It is important to diagnose and treat these conditions early, as they are associated with poor prognosis and high mortality.
- The pathophysiology underlying these complex cardiorenal interactions requires a thorough understanding of both traditional and nontraditional risk factors.
- Management of patients with cardiorenal syndromes can be complicated owing to limitations of diagnostic and therapeutic modalities.
- Although several established and novel therapeutic targets are being increasingly used to optimize management of this population, there remains a paucity of data from large cardiovascular trials owing to underrepresentation of these high-risk patients.

DISCLOSURE

Dr A. Spirito received a research grant from the Swiss National Science Foundation (SNSF). Dr R. Mehran reports institutional research grants from Abbott, Abiomed, Applied Therapeutics, Arena, AstraZeneca, Bayer, Biosensors, Boston Scientific, Bristol-Myers Squibb, CardiaWave, CellAegis, CERC, Chiesi, Concept Medical, CSL Behring, DSI, Insel Gruppe AG, Medtronic, Novartis Pharmaceuticals, OrbusNeich, Philips, Transverse Medical, Zoll; personal fees from ACC, Boston Scientific, California Institute for Regenerative Medicine (CIRM), Cine-Med Research, Janssen, WebMD, SCAI; consulting fees paid to the institution from Abbott, Abiomed, AM-Pharma, Alleviant Medical, Bayer, Beth Israel Deaconess, CardiaWave, CeloNova, Chiesi, Concept Medical, DSI, Duke University, Idorsia Pharmaceuticals, Medtronic, Novartis, Philips; Equity <1% in Applied Therapeutics, Elixir Medical, STEL, CONTROLRAD (spouse); Scientific Advisory Board for AMA, Biosensors (spouse). The remaining authors have nothing to disclose.

REFERENCES

1. Bright R. Cases and observations illustrative of renal disease accompanied with the secretion of albuminous urine. Guy's Hospital Report 1836; 10:338–40.

2. Rangaswami J, Bhalla V, Blair JEA, et al. Cardiore-nal Syndrome: Classification, Pathophysiology, Diagnosis, and Treatment Strategies: A Scientific Statement From the American Heart Association. Circulation 2019;139(16):e840–78.

3. House AA, Anand I, Bellomo R, et al. Definition and classification of Cardio-Renal Syndromes: workgroup statements from the 7th ADQI Consensus Conference. Nephrol Dial Transplant 2010;25(5):1416–20.

4. Heywood JT. The cardiorenal syndrome: lessons from the ADHERE database and treatment op-tions. Heart Fail Rev 2004;9(3):195–201.

5. Global, regional, and national burden of chronic kidney disease, 1990-2017: a systematic analysis for the Global Burden of Disease Study 2017. Lan-cet 2020;395(10225):709–33.

6. Global, regional, and national incidence, preva-lence, and years lived with disability for 354 dis-eases and injuries for 195 countries and territories, 1990-2017: a systematic analysis for the Global Burden of Disease Study 2017. Lancet 2018;392(10159):1789–858.

7. Stevens PE, O'Donoghue DJ, de Lusignan S, et al. Chronic kidney disease management in the United Kingdom: NEOERICA project results. Kid-ney Int 2007;72(1):92–9.

8. Ezekowitz J, McAlister FA, Humphries KH, et al. The association among renal insufficiency, phar-macotherapy, and outcomes in 6,427 patients with heart failure and coronary artery disease. J Am Coll Cardiol 2004;44(8):1587–92.

9. Damman K, Valente MA, Voors AA, et al. Renal impairment, worsening renal function, and outcome in patients with heart failure: an updated meta-analysis. Eur Heart J 2014;35(7):455–69.

10. Tonelli M, Wiebe N, Culleton B, et al. Chronic kid-ney disease and mortality risk: a systematic re-view. J Am Soc Nephrol 2006;17(7):2034–47.

11. Thompson S, James M, Wiebe N, et al. Cause of Death in Patients with Reduced Kidney Function. J Am Soc Nephrol 2015;26(10):2504–11.

12. Webster AC, Nagler EV, Morton RL, et al. Chronic Kidney Disease. Lancet 2017;389(10075):1238–52.

13. Ronco C, McCullough P, Anker SD, et al. Cardio-renal syndromes: report from the consensus con-ference of the acute dialysis quality initiative. Eur Heart J 2010;31(6):703–11.

14. Mavrakanas TA, Khattak A, Singh K, et al. Epide-miology and Natural History of the Cardiorenal Syndromes in a Cohort with Echocardiography. Clin J Am Soc Nephrol 2017;12(10):1624–33.

15. Major RW, Cheng MRI, Grant RA, et al. Cardiovas-cular disease risk factors in chronic kidney disease: A systematic review and meta-analysis. PLoS One 2018;13(3):e0192895.

16. Wilson PW, D'Agostino RB, Levy D, et al. Pre-diction of coronary heart disease using risk factor categories. Circulation 1998;97(18):1837–47.

17. Centers for Disease Control and Prevention. Chronic kidney disease in the United States, 2021. Atlanta, GA: US Department of Health and Human Services, Centers for Disease Control and Prevention; 2021.

18. Roehm B, Weiner DE. Blood pressure targets and kidney and cardiovascular disease: same data but discordant guidelines. Curr Opin Nephrol Hyper-tens 2019;28(3):245–50.

19. Di Lullo L, Reeves PB, Bellasi A, et al. Cardiorenal Syndrome in Acute Kidney Injury. Semin Nephrol 2019;39(1):31–40.

20. Long DA, Price KL, Herrera-Acosta J, et al. How does angiotensin II cause renal injury? Hyperten-sion 2004;43(4):722–3.

21. Giam B, Kaye DM, Rajapakse NW. Role of Renal Oxidative Stress in the Pathogenesis of the Cardi-orenal Syndrome. Heart Lung Circ 2016;25(8):874–80.

22. Raina R, Nair N, Chakraborty R, et al. An Update on the Pathophysiology and Treatment of Cardi-orenal Syndrome. Cardiol Res 2020;11(2):76–88.

23. Wu J, You J, Wang S, et al. Insights Into the Acti-vation and Inhibition of Angiotensin II Type 1 Re-ceptor in the Mechanically Loaded Heart. Circ J 2014;78(6):1283–9.

24. Zhu Y-C, Zhu Y-Z, Gohlke P, et al. Effects of Angiotensin-Converting Enzyme Inhibition and Angiotensin II AT$_1$ Receptor Antagonism on Car-diac Parameters in Left Ventricular Hypertrophy. Am J Cardiol 1997;80(3). 110A-7A.

25. Diniz GP, Carneiro-Ramos MS, Barreto-Chaves MLM. Angiotensin type 1 receptor medi-ates thyroid hormone-induced cardiomyocyte hypertrophy through the Akt/GSK-3β/mTOR signaling pathway. Basic Res Cardiol 2009;104(6):653–67.

26. Vignier N, Le Corvoisier P, Blard C, et al. AT1 blockade abolishes left ventricular hypertrophy in heterozygous cMyBP-C null mice: role of FHL1. Fund Clin Pharmacol 2014;28(3):249–56.

27. Patel A, MacMahon S, Chalmers J, et al. Intensive blood glucose control and vascular outcomes in patients with type 2 diabetes. N Engl J Med 2008;358(24):2560–72.

28. Zewinger S, Kleber ME, Rohrer L, et al. Symmetric dimethylarginine, high-density lipoproteins and cardiovascular disease. Eur Heart J 2017;38(20):1597–607.

29. Shroff R, Speer T, Colin S, et al. HDL in children with CKD promotes endothelial dysfunction and an abnormal vascular phenotype. J Am Soc Neph-rol 2014;25(11):2658–68.

30. Patel B, Ismahil MA, Hamid T, et al. Mononuclear Phagocytes Are Dispensable for Cardiac Remodeling in Established Pressure-Overload Heart Failure. PLoS One 2017;12(1):e0170781.

31. Savira F, Magaye R, Liew D, et al. Cardiorenal syndrome: Multi-organ dysfunction involving the heart, kidney and vasculature. Br J Pharmacol 2020;177(13):2906–22.

32. Ridker PM, MacFadyen JG, Glynn RJ, et al. Inhibition of Interleukin-1β by Canakinumab and Cardiovascular Outcomes in Patients With Chronic Kidney Disease. J Am Coll Cardiol 2018;71(21):2405–14.

33. Chen B, Frangogiannis NG. Immune cells in repair of the infarcted myocardium. Microcirculation 2017;24(1):e12305.

34. Clementi A, Virzì GM, Brocca A, et al. Advances in the pathogenesis of cardiorenal syndrome type 3. Oxidative medicine and cellular Longevity, 2015, 2015. p. 148082.

35. Brunet P, Gondouin B, Duval-Sabatier A, et al. Does Uremia Cause Vascular Dysfunction. Kidney Blood Press Res 2011;34(4):284–90.

36. Chaudhary K, Malhotra K, Sowers J, et al. Uric Acid - Key Ingredient in the Recipe for Cardiorenal Metabolic Syndrome. Cardiorenal Med 2013;3(3):208–20.

37. Lekawanvijit S. Cardiotoxicity of Uremic Toxins: A Driver of Cardiorenal Syndrome. Toxins 2018;10(9):352.

38. Wu IW, Hsu KH, Lee CC, et al. p-Cresyl sulphate and indoxyl sulphate predict progression of chronic kidney disease. Nephrol Dial Transplant 2011;26(3):938–47.

39. Dhingra R, Gona P, Benjamin EJ, et al. Relations of serum phosphorus levels to echocardiographic left ventricular mass and incidence of heart failure in the community. Eur J Heart Fail 2010;12(8):812–8.

40. Tonelli M, Sacks F, Pfeffer M, et al. Relation Between Serum Phosphate Level and Cardiovascular Event Rate in People With Coronary Disease. Circulation 2005;112(17):2627–33.

41. Faul C, Amaral AP, Oskouei B, et al. FGF23 induces left ventricular hypertrophy. J Clin Investig 2011;121(11):4393–408.

42. Navarro-García JA, Delgado C, Fernández-Velasco M, et al. Fibroblast growth factor-23 promotes rhythm alterations and contractile dysfunction in adult ventricular cardiomyocytes. Nephrol Dial Transplant 2019;34(11):1864–75.

43. Gaikwad AB, Sayyed SG, Lichtnekert J, et al. Renal Failure Increases Cardiac Histone H3 Acetylation, Dimethylation, and Phosphorylation and the Induction of Cardiomyopathy-Related Genes in Type 2 Diabetes. Am J Pathol 2010;176(3):1079–83.

44. Huang C-K, Bär C, Thum T. miR-21, Mediator, and Potential Therapeutic Target in the Cardiorenal Syndrome. Front Pharmacol 2020;11.

45. Thum T, Gross C, Fiedler J, et al. MicroRNA-21 contributes to myocardial disease by stimulating MAP kinase signalling in fibroblasts. Nature 2008;456(7224):980–4.

46. Monroy MA, Fang J, Li S, et al. Chronic kidney disease alters vascular smooth muscle cell phenotype. Front Biosci (Landmark Ed) 2015;20(4):784–95.

47. Dube P, DeRiso A, Patel M, et al. Vascular Calcification in Chronic Kidney Disease: Diversity in the Vessel Wall. Biomedicines 2021;9(4).

48. Ureña-Torres P, D'Marco L, Raggi P, et al. Valvular heart disease and calcification in CKD: more common than appreciated. Nephrol Dial Transplant 2020;35(12):2046–53.

49. O'Neill WC, Lomashvili KA. Recent progress in the treatment of vascular calcification. Kidney Int 2010;78(12):1232–9.

50. Goodman WG, Goldin J, Kuizon BD, et al. Coronary-artery calcification in young adults with end-stage renal disease who are undergoing dialysis. N Engl J Med 2000;342(20):1478–83.

51. Guérin AP, London GM, Marchais SJ, et al. Arterial stiffening and vascular calcifications in end-stage renal disease. Nephrol Dial Transplant 2000;15(7):1014–21.

52. Shobeiri N, Pang J, Adams MA, et al. Cardiovascular disease in an adenine-induced model of chronic kidney disease: the temporal link between vascular calcification and haemodynamic consequences. J Hypertens 2013;31(1):160–8.

53. Brandenburg VM, Schuh A, Kramann R. Valvular Calcification in Chronic Kidney Disease. Adv Chronic Kidney Dis 2019;26(6):464–71.

54. Di Lullo L, Gorini A, Russo D, et al. Left Ventricular Hypertrophy in Chronic Kidney Disease Patients: From Pathophysiology to Treatment. Cardiorenal Med 2015;5(4):254–66.

55. Konstantinidis I, Nadkarni GN, Yacoub R, et al. Representation of Patients With Kidney Disease in Trials of Cardiovascular Interventions: An Updated Systematic Review. JAMA Intern Med 2016;176(1):121–4.

56. Wanner C, Amann K, Shoji T. The heart and vascular system in dialysis. Lancet 2016;388(10041):276–84.

57. Wang LW, Fahim MA, Hayen A, et al. Cardiac testing for coronary artery disease in potential kidney transplant recipients: a systematic review of test accuracy studies. Am J Kidney Dis 2011;57(3):476–87.

58. Sarnak MJ, Amann K, Bangalore S, et al. Chronic Kidney Disease and Coronary Artery Disease:

JACC State-of-the-Art Review. J Am Coll Cardiol 2019;74(14):1823–38.

59. Winther S, Svensson M, Jørgensen HS, et al. Diagnostic Performance of Coronary CT Angiography and Myocardial Perfusion Imaging in Kidney Transplantation Candidates. JACC Cardiovasc Imaging 2015;8(5):553–62.

60. Al-Mallah MH, Hachamovitch R, Dorbala S, et al. Incremental prognostic value of myocardial perfusion imaging in patients referred to stress single-photon emission computed tomography with renal dysfunction. Circ Cardiovasc Imaging 2009; 2(6):429–36.

61. Breidthardt T, Burton JO, Odudu A, et al. Troponin T for the detection of dialysis-induced myocardial stunning in hemodialysis patients. Clin J Am Soc Nephrol 2012;7(8):1285–92.

62. Dionísio LM, Luvizoto MJ, Gribner C, et al. Biomarkers of cardio-renal syndrome in uremic myocardiopathy animal model. J Bras Nefrol 2018; 40(2):105–11.

63. KDIGO 2021 Clinical Practice Guideline for the Management of Blood Pressure in Chronic Kidney Disease. Kidney Int 2021;99(3s):S1–s87.

64. Visseren FLJ, Mach F, Smulders YM, et al. ESC Guidelines on cardiovascular disease prevention in clinical practice. Eur Heart J 2021;42(34):3227–337.

65. Kollias A, Kyriakoulis KG, Stergiou GS. Blood pressure target for hypertension in chronic kidney disease: One size does not fit all. J Clin Hypertens 2020;22(5):929–32.

66. Ismail-Beigi F, Craven T, Banerji MA, et al. Effect of intensive treatment of hyperglycaemia on microvascular outcomes in type 2 diabetes: an analysis of the ACCORD randomised trial. Lancet 2010;376(9739):419–30.

67. Intensive blood-glucose control with sulphonylureas or insulin compared with conventional treatment and risk of complications in patients with type 2 diabetes (UKPDS 33). UK Prospective Diabetes Study (UKPDS) Group. Lancet 1998; 352(9131):837–53.

68. Zoungas S, Chalmers J, Neal B, et al. Follow-up of blood-pressure lowering and glucose control in type 2 diabetes. N Engl J Med 2014;371(15): 1392–406.

69. Hemmingsen B, Lund SS, Gluud C, et al. Targeting intensive glycaemic control versus targeting conventional glycaemic control for type 2 diabetes mellitus. Cochrane Database Syst Rev 2013;(11):Cd008143.

70. Wanner C. EMPA-REG OUTCOME: The Nephrologist's Point of View. Am J Cardiol 2017;120(1): S59–67.

71. Marso SP, Daniels GH, Brown-Frandsen K, et al. Liraglutide and Cardiovascular Outcomes in Type 2 Diabetes. N Engl J Med 2016;375(4): 311–22.

72. Marso SP, Bain SC, Consoli A, et al. Semaglutide and Cardiovascular Outcomes in Patients with Type 2 Diabetes. N Engl J Med 2016;375(19): 1834–44.

73. Gerstein HC, Colhoun HM, Dagenais GR, et al. Dulaglutide and cardiovascular outcomes in type 2 diabetes (REWIND): a double-blind, randomised placebo-controlled trial. Lancet 2019;394(10193): 121–30.

74. Baigent C, Landray MJ, Reith C, et al. The effects of lowering LDL cholesterol with simvastatin plus ezetimibe in patients with chronic kidney disease (Study of Heart and Renal Protection): a randomised placebo-controlled trial. Lancet 2011; 377(9784):2181–92.

75. Wanner C, Krane V, März W, et al. Atorvastatin in patients with type 2 diabetes mellitus undergoing hemodialysis. N Engl J Med 2005;353(3): 238–48.

76. Fellström BC, Jardine AG, Schmieder RE, et al. Rosuvastatin and cardiovascular events in patients undergoing hemodialysis. N Engl J Med 2009; 360(14):1395–407.

77. Charytan DM, Sabatine MS, Pedersen TR, et al. Efficacy and Safety of Evolocumab in Chronic Kidney Disease in the FOURIER Trial. J Am Coll Cardiol 2019;73(23):2961–70.

78. Palmer SC, Di Micco L, Razavian M, et al. Antiplatelet agents for chronic kidney disease. Cochrane Database Syst Rev 2013;(2): Cd008834.

79. Costa F, van Klaveren D, James S, et al. Derivation and validation of the predicting bleeding complications in patients undergoing stent implantation and subsequent dual antiplatelet therapy (PRECISE-DAPT) score: a pooled analysis of individual-patient datasets from clinical trials. Lancet 2017;389(10073):1025–34.

80. Yeh RW, Secemsky EA, Kereiakes DJ, et al. Development and Validation of a Prediction Rule for Benefit and Harm of Dual Antiplatelet Therapy Beyond 1 Year After Percutaneous Coronary Intervention. JAMA 2016;315(16):1735–49.

81. Urban P, Mehran R, Colleran R, et al. Defining High Bleeding Risk in Patients Undergoing Percutaneous Coronary Intervention. Circulation 2019; 140(3):240–61.

82. Charytan DM, Wallentin L, Lagerqvist B, et al. Early angiography in patients with chronic kidney disease: a collaborative systematic review. Clin J Am Soc Nephrol 2009;4(6):1032–43.

83. Bangalore S, Maron DJ, O'Brien SM, et al. Management of Coronary Disease in Patients with Advanced Kidney Disease. N Engl J Med 2020; 382(17):1608–18.

84. Chandiramani R, Cao D, Nicolas J, et al. Contrast-induced acute kidney injury. Cardiovasc Interv Ther 2020;35(3):209–17.

85. Ghali JK, Wikstrand J, Van Veldhuisen DJ, et al. The influence of renal function on clinical outcome and response to beta-blockade in systolic heart failure: insights from Metoprolol CR/XL Randomized Intervention Trial in Chronic HF (MERIT-HF). J Card Fail 2009;15(4):310–8.

86. Badve SV, Roberts MA, Hawley CM, et al. Effects of beta-adrenergic antagonists in patients with chronic kidney disease: a systematic review and meta-analysis. J Am Coll Cardiol 2011;58(11):1152–61.

87. Ahmed A, Fonarow GC, Zhang Y, et al. Renin-angiotensin inhibition in systolic heart failure and chronic kidney disease. Am J Med 2012;125(4):399–410.

88. Baudrand R, Guarda FJ, Fardella C, et al. Continuum of Renin-Independent Aldosteronism in Normotension. Hypertension 2017;69(5):950–6.

89. Navaneethan SD, Nigwekar SU, Sehgal AR, et al. Aldosterone antagonists for preventing the progression of chronic kidney disease: a systematic review and meta-analysis. Clin J Am Soc Nephrol 2009;4(3):542–51.

90. Pitt B, Zannad F, Remme WJ, et al. The effect of spironolactone on morbidity and mortality in patients with severe heart failure. Randomized Aldactone Evaluation Study Investigators. N Engl J Med 1999;341(10):709–17.

91. Zannad F, McMurray JJ, Krum H, et al. Eplerenone in patients with systolic heart failure and mild symptoms. N Engl J Med 2011;364(1):11–21.

92. Bakris GL, Agarwal R, Anker SD, et al. Effect of Finerenone on Chronic Kidney Disease Outcomes in Type 2 Diabetes. N Engl J Med 2020;383(23):2219–29.

93. Hammer F, Malzahn U, Donhauser J, et al. A randomized controlled trial of the effect of spironolactone on left ventricular mass in hemodialysis patients. Kidney Int 2019;95(4):983–91.

94. Charytan DM, Himmelfarb J, Ikizler TA, et al. Safety and cardiovascular efficacy of spironolactone in dialysis-dependent ESRD (SPin-D): a randomized, placebo-controlled, multiple dosage trial. Kidney Int 2019;95(4):973–82.

95. Klein L, Massie BM, Leimberger JD, et al. Admission or changes in renal function during hospitalization for worsening heart failure predict postdischarge survival: results from the Outcomes of a Prospective Trial of Intravenous Milrinone for Exacerbations of Chronic Heart Failure (OPTIME-CHF). Circ Heart Fail 2008;1(1):25–33.

96. Giamouzis G, Butler J, Starling RC, et al. Impact of dopamine infusion on renal function in hospitalized heart failure patients: results of the Dopamine in Acute Decompensated Heart Failure (DAD-HF) Trial. J Card Fail 2010;16(12):922–30.

97. Mullens W, Abrahams Z, Francis GS, et al. Sodium nitroprusside for advanced low-output heart failure. J Am Coll Cardiol 2008;52(3):200–7.

98. Kim CS. Pharmacologic Management of the Cardio-renal Syndrome. Electrolyte Blood Press 2013;11(1):17–23.

99. Massie BM, O'Connor CM, Metra M, et al. Rolofylline, an adenosine A1-receptor antagonist, in acute heart failure. N Engl J Med 2010;363(15):1419–28.

100. Packer M, Anker SD, Butler J, et al. Cardiovascular and Renal Outcomes with Empagliflozin in Heart Failure. N Engl J Med 2020;383(15):1413–24.

101. Anker SD, Butler J, Filippatos G, et al. Empagliflozin in Heart Failure with a Preserved Ejection Fraction. N Engl J Med 2021;385(16):1451–61.

102. McGuire DK, Shih WJ, Cosentino F, et al. Association of SGLT2 Inhibitors With Cardiovascular and Kidney Outcomes in Patients With Type 2 Diabetes: A Meta-analysis. JAMA Cardiology 2021;6(2):148–58.

103. Costanzo MR, Guglin ME, Saltzberg MT, et al. Ultrafiltration versus intravenous diuretics for patients hospitalized for acute decompensated heart failure. J Am Coll Cardiol 2007;49(6):675–83.

104. Bart BA, Goldsmith SR, Lee KL, et al. Ultrafiltration in decompensated heart failure with cardiorenal syndrome. N Engl J Med 2012;367(24):2296–304.

105. Costanzo MR, Negoianu D, Jaski BE, et al. Aquapheresis Versus Intravenous Diuretics and Hospitalizations for Heart Failure. JACC Heart Fail 2016;4(2):95–105.

106. Genovesi S, Boriani G, Covic A, et al. Sudden cardiac death in dialysis patients: different causes and management strategies. Nephrol Dial Transplant 2021;36(3):396–405.

107. Perl J, Chan CT. Timing of sudden death relative to the hemodialysis procedure. Nat Clin Pract Nephrol 2006;2(12):668–9.

108. Korantzopoulos P, Liu T, Li L, et al. Implantable cardioverter defibrillator therapy in chronic kidney disease: a meta-analysis. Europace 2009;11(11):1469–75.

109. Wong MC, Kalman JM, Pedagogos E, et al. Temporal distribution of arrhythmic events in chronic kidney disease: Highest incidence in the long interdialytic period. Heart Rhythm 2015;12(10):2047–55.

110. Sacher F, Jesel L, Borni-Duval C, et al. Cardiac Rhythm Disturbances in Hemodialysis Patients: Early Detection Using an Implantable Loop Recorder and Correlation With Biological and Dialysis Parameters. JACC Clin Electrophysiol 2018;4(3):397–408.

111. Ifedili IA, Bolorunduro O, Bob-Manuel T, et al. Impact of Pre-existing Kidney Dysfunction on Outcomes Following Transcatheter Aortic Valve Replacement. Curr Cardiol Rev 2017;13(4): 283–92.

112. Fernando M, Paterson HS, Byth K, et al. Outcomes of cardiac surgery in chronic kidney disease. J Thorac Cardiovasc Surg 2014;148(5): 2167–73.

113. Baumgartner H, Falk V, Bax JJ, et al. ESC/EACTS Guidelines for the management of valvular heart disease. Eur Heart J 2017;38(36): 2739–91.

114. Popma JJ, Deeb GM, Yakubov SJ, et al. Transcatheter Aortic-Valve Replacement with a Self-Expanding Valve in Low-Risk Patients. N Engl J Med 2019;380(18):1706–15.

115. Mack MJ, Leon MB, Thourani VH, et al. Transcatheter Aortic-Valve Replacement with a Balloon-Expandable Valve in Low-Risk Patients. N Engl J Med 2019;380(18):1695–705.

116. Doshi R, Shlofmitz E, Shah J, et al. Comparison of Transcatheter Mitral Valve Repair Versus Surgical Mitral Valve Repair in Patients With Advanced Kidney Disease (from the National Inpatient Sample). Am J Cardiol 2018;121(6):762–7.

117. Shah B, Vemulapalli S, Manandhar P, et al. OUTCOMES AFTER TRANSCATHETER MITRAL VALVE REPAIR IN PATIENTS WITH CHRONIC KIDNEY DISEASE: AN ANALYSIS OF 5,241 PATIENTS IN THE UNITED STATES. J Am Coll Cardiol 2018;71(11_Supplement):A1980–.

118. Shalhoub V, Shatzen EM, Ward SC, et al. FGF23 neutralization improves chronic kidney disease-associated hyperparathyroidism yet increases mortality. J Clin Invest 2012;122(7):2543–53.

119. Leifheit-Nestler M, Grabner A, Hermann L, et al. Vitamin D treatment attenuates cardiac FGF23/FGFR4 signaling and hypertrophy in uremic rats. Nephrol Dial Transplant 2017;32(9):1493–503.

120. Alarcon MML, Trentin-Sonoda M, Panico K, et al. Cardiac arrhythmias after renal I/R depend on IL-1β. Journal of Molecular and Cellular Cardiology 2019;131:101–11.

121. Monnerat G, Alarcón ML, Vasconcellos LR, et al. Macrophage-dependent IL-1β production induces cardiac arrhythmias in diabetic mice. Nat Commun 2016;7(1):13344.

Definition, Staging, and Role of Biomarkers in Acute Kidney Injury in the Context of Cardiovascular Interventions

Prakash S. Gudsoorkar, MD[a,b,*], Jacob Nysather, MD[a,b],
Charuhas V. Thakar, MD[a,b,c]

KEYWORDS

- Acute kidney injury (AKI) • Biomarkers • Cardiac surgery • Cardiorenal syndrome
- Contrast associated AKI

KEY POINTS

- Changes in the serum creatinine and urine output have been used to define acute kidney injury (AKI), and the criteria have evolved over time with better understanding of the impact of AKI on the outcomes.
- Reliance on serum creatinine for these AKI definitions carries numerous limitations including delayed rise, inability to differentiate between hemodynamics versus structural injury and assay variability to name a few.
- Novel biomarkers have been proposed and investigated to overcome these limitations and capture the real AKI events.

INTRODUCTION

Acute kidney injury (AKI) is a frequent and sometimes devastating syndrome in patients undergoing cardiovascular interventions. It has multiple risk factors or causes and has been reported to occur in up to 7% to 30% patients depending on the intervention and clinical scenario, with high costs to patients and health care systems. Therefore, a uniform definition of AKI is needed that can be applied in both clinical practice and research to enable timely recognition and treatment consistently across health care systems. Definition of AKI has evolved over the years, with an increased understanding of different etiologies and the integration of novel biomarkers to improve predictive and preventative strategies to enhance outcomes. This article reviews the evolution of defining AKI and how the cardiology community has adopted and modified these definitions. This review also explores the pitfalls associated with defining AKI, its impact on diagnoses and outcomes, and the application of biomarkers in various cardiovascular interventions and clinical scenarios.

DEFINITIONS OF ACUTE KIDNEY INJURY

Defining AKI had been challenging due to variations in criteria used in earlier studies, making data comparison difficult. In 2004, the Acute Disease Quality Initiative (ADQI) introduced standardized RIFLE criteria (Risk, Injury, Failure, Loss of kidney function, End-stage kidney disease).[1] The AKI definition continued to evolve with the introduction of AKI-Network (AKIN)

[a] Division of Nephrology and Kidney CARE Program, Department of Medicine, University of Cincinnati, OH, USA;
[b] Division of Nephrology and Kidney Clinical Advancement, Research & Education (C.A.R.E.) Program, University of Cincinnati, 231 Albert Sabin Way, OH 45267, USA; [c] Department of Nephrology, Veterans Administration Medical Center, Cincinnati, OH, USA
* Corresponding author. Division of Nephrology and Kidney Clinical Advancement, Research & Education (C.A.R.E.) Program, University of Cincinnati, 231 Albert Sabin Way, OH 45267.
E-mail address: GUDSOOPS@ucmail.uc.edu

Intervent Cardiol Clin 12 (2023) 469–487
https://doi.org/10.1016/j.iccl.2023.06.004

criteria and, most recently, Kidney Disease: Improving Global Outcomes (KDIGO) criteria in nephrology literature.[2] This evolution in definition has been driven by the need to improve accuracy and consistency in the diagnosis and management of AKI. The latest KDIGO criteria define AKI as rise in serum creatinine (SCr) by $\geq$ 0.3 mg/dL within 48 hours or greater than or equal to 50% within 7 days. These criteria increase both sensitivity and specificity for a meaningful AKI (Table 1).

Because of complexity and increase in mortality, AKI is a quality metric for in-hospital cardiovascular procedures in the United States and is recorded through numerous outcome registries. One of these associations is the Valve Academic Research Consortium (VARC) for heart valve procedures such as transcatheter aortic valve replacement (TAVR). The definition of AKI has been modified by VARC based on adaptations and further updates within the council for monitoring outcomes: 2011 VARC-1, 2014 VARC-2, and 2021 VARC-3 are adaptations of RIFLE,[3] AKIN criteria,[4] KDIGO criteria,[5] respectively. The latest VARC-3 adopts KDIGO criteria however excludes urine output due to its challenges in the clinical practice and separates the need for renal replacement therapy (RRT) as stage IV AKI. Nonetheless, many in the cardiovascular community including ACC-NCDR (American College of Cardiology National Cardiovascular Data Registry), CathPCI (percutaneous coronary interventions),[6,7] ACC-NCDR PVI (peripheral vascular interventions),[8,9] and Society of Thoracic Surgery–Transcatheter Valve Therapy (STS-TVT) continue to use the AKIN framework.[10] A Scientific Workshop cosponsored by the National Kidney Foundation and the Society for Cardiovascular Angiography and Interventions writing committee suggests adopting the KDIGO criteria to define AKI for future studies in the context of cardiovascular procedures.[11]

Studies have directly compared these definitions of AKI to assess the impact on outcomes; however, most of these studies included patient population sustaining AKI due to sepsis, liver failure or in intensive care units, hospitalized and pediatric patients; very few studies have compared these definitions within cardiovascular intervention literature. In a study by Koifman and colleagues, in 217 patients undergoing TAVR, AKI occurred in 23% and 21% of patients according to VARC-2 and RIFLE definitions, respectively, with an approximate 10% disagreement between both systems. AKI defined by either classification was independently associated with 2-year mortality (hazard ratio [HR] 1.63, for the VARC-2 definition and HR 1.60 for RIFLE definition, P-value = 0.04 for both), with borderline superiority of the VARC-2 classification.[12]

There are no comparative studies between VARC and KDIGO definition, which have a very subtle difference in the AKI stage 1 criteria (see Table 1). Evaluation of AKI incidence by subpopulations (eg, presence of chronic kidney disease [CKD] stage, age, etc.) may explain some of the differences observed between studies. Sutherland and colleagues[13] compared these definitions in patients undergoing cardiac surgeries (coronary artery bypass graft, heart/lung transplantation, valve repair/replacements, aortic surgery, and others). KDIGO definition was the most sensitive in identifying AKI; however, it diagnosed some patients with AKI that might not have been clinically relevant. On the contrary, AKIN criteria missed up to 17% diagnosed by the other criteria.[13] In this study, a subset of the patients had a slow increase in SCr described as "late AKI" (defined as > 0.3 mg/dL increase in SCr >72 hours after intervention). These were labeled "missed AKIs" but would fall under subclinical AKI or acute kidney disease (AKD) definitions. This study, however, did not include urine output criteria. Similar findings between criteria are noted with acute decompensated heart failure (ADHF).[14] Overall, these trends are identical to what have been encountered in other noncardiac patient populations and highlights the limitations of these definitions.

PITFALLS TO CONSIDER WHEN DEFINING ACUTE KIDNEY INJURY BASED ON SERUM CREATININE AND URINE OUTPUT

Many pitfalls were noted with increased use of earlier definitions, and attempts have been made to address these limitations in the modern modifications. For example, omission of "loss" and "end-stage"' stages from RIFLE criteria that represent outcomes than the stages of AKI. Glomerular filtration rate (GFR) was included in the original RIFLE criteria; however, for AKI, GFR use is inappropriate primarily due to lack of steady state[15] leading to removal of GFR in subsequent guidelines. AKIN criteria required adequate fluid resuscitation and urinary obstruction to be excluded before applying serum creatinine criteria. Hypovolemia and obstruction have their own implication on the outcomes; hence, the latest KDIGO did not include these specifications to define AKI.[2]

Oliguria results from interaction of complex pathophysiologic processes with many variables

Table 1
Definitions and staging of acute kidney injury

Nephrology	RIFLE[b] (2004)[1]	AKIN (2007)[2]	KDIGO (2012)	Urine Output Criteria[a]
Definition of AKI	–	Increase by ≥ 0.3 mg/dL or ≥50% within 48 h	Increased by ≥ 0.3 mg/dL within 48 h or ≥50% within 7 d	< 0.5 mL/kg/h for ≥6 h
Stage 1/risk	Increased by ≥ 1.5 times baseline; or decrease in GFR by ≥ 25%	Increased by ≥ 0.3 mg/dL or 1.5–2.0 times baseline	Increased by ≥ 0.3 mg/dL or 1.5–1.9 times baseline	< 0.5 mL/kg/h for 6–12 h
Stage 2/injury	Increased by ≥ 2.0 times baseline; or decrease in GFR by ≥ 50%	Increased by > 2.0 to 3.0 times baseline	Increased by 2.0–2.9 times baseline	< 0.5 mL/kg/h for ≥12 h
Stage 3/failure	Increased by ≥ 3.0 times baseline; or > 0.5 mg/dL to > 4.0 mg/dL; or decrease in GFR by ≥ 75%	Increased by > 3 times baseline; or ≥0.5 mg/dL to ≥4.0 mg/dL; or on KRT	Increased ≥ 3.0 times baseline; or ≥0.3 mg/dL to ≥4.0 mg/dL; or on KRT	< 0.3 mL/kg/h for ≥24 h; or anuria for ≥12 h
RIFLE Loss	KRT dependent for > 4 wk	–	–	–
RIFLE End-stage	KRT dependent of > 3 mo	–	–	–
Cardiology:	VARC-1 (2011)	VARC-2 (2012)	VARC-3 (2021)	
Modifications	Re-classification as stages 1–3; removal of RIFLE L and E; change of ≥0.3 mg/dL; introduction of <72 h from index procedure. KRT automatically designated as stage 3	Serum creatinine change of ≥0.3 mg/dL up to 72 h post-procedure, with % change from baseline extended to 7 d	Separation of those requiring KRT and classifying these as stage 4, excluding ESKD	Not included in VARC definitions[c]

AKIN: Acute Kidney Injury Network; ESKD: end stage kidney disease; KDIGO: Kidney Disease Improving Global Outcomes; KRT: kidney replacement therapy; RIFLE: Risk, Injury, Failure, Loss, End-stage classification; VARC: Valve Academic Research Consortium

[a] Urine output criteria are identical for the RIFLE, AKIN, and KDIGO criteria.
[b] Rather than a single definition and staging categories, the RIFLE classification provided definitions of AKI with increasing stringency but decreasing sensitivity (risk, injury, and failure) and 2 outcome categories based on the duration of KRT-dependence (loss and end-stage disease).
[c] Each VARC criteria omit urine output in defining AKI given practical challenges in accuracy and routine collection for measurement. Staging of AKI is based solely on serum creatinine. Urine output may be used in context of a designated AKI study.

not only hemodynamic changes or tubular necrosis.[16] These factors include fluid balance, diuretic use, and differing weights (actual, idea, or lean body mass) that can affect weight-based definitions of urine output. Oliguria with or without rise in creatinine independently predicts a higher risk of mortality.[17] Oliguria is typically defined as urine output less than 0.5 mL/kg/h for 6 consecutive hours.[1,2] However, a threshold of less than 0.3 mL/kg/h for 6 hours demonstrated the best predictive of mortality and/or need for dialysis suggesting that the current criterion is too liberal.[18] Shorter durations (<4 hours) of oliguria is associated with reduced sensitivity and specificity in predicting AKI.[19] Nonetheless, the existing urine output criteria identify a higher percentage of patients with AKI compared with SCr criteria alone.[20] However, it may not translate into predicting improved mortality and may have different prognostic implications depending on AKI etiologies; thus, it requires further investigation.[21]

In clinical practice, the small changes in SCr (increase of $\geq$ 0.3 mg/dL representing stage I AKI) are often attributed to intra-assay laboratory variations. This criterion of minor change in SCr takes into account of lab variations while maintaining sensitivity to diagnose AKI. The modern analyzers are very accurate and increments of 0.3 mg/dL are unlikely due to assay variation.[22] There are still concerns of overly sensitive results with increased false positive results with these small increments. Nevertheless, these small changes occur frequently and have been independently associated with increased mortality.[23]

Acute injury in CKD represents a population not previously included in early guidelines. Percentage rises in creatinine are curtailed in CKD and do not readily detect acute on CKD. It is known that progressively larger absolute rises in creatinine are required to show an independent association with mortality as the baseline GFR falls. Current AKI staging may have lower prognostic value in CKD when based on absolute increases in creatinine at the lower end of the spectrum. However, given the serious risk CKD patients face, KDIGO addresses this subgroup with modification to stage 3 criteria as any rise in SCr to greater than 4.0 mg/dL, even when the rise in SCr greater than or equal to 0.3 mg/dL or greater than 50% change. In contrast, similar changes without CKD are classified as stage 1.[21] Limitations of SCr as a biomarker are discussed separately below.

The time constraint of 48 hours was selected based upon evidence of adverse outcomes with small changes observed within that time frame and a maximum time for changes up to 7 days following events.[24–26] By incorporating a specific time frame into the AKIN and other similar definitions, the intention is to exclude those elevations in SCr without acute injury.[2] Further, the population that does not meet the criteria for AKI within time designation but exhibits impairment (subclinical AKI) outside of the specified time frame is described as Acute Kidney Disease by the 2020 KDIGO Consensus Conference.[27]

Role of biomarkers
Limitation serum creatinine-based criteria
The current standards of care used in diagnosing AKI have several limitations. SCr and urine output changes become apparent several hours to days after a significant decline in GFR. The rise in SCr can also represent a functional (reversible) change, not necessarily a structural injury to the nephron. Also, it does not provide any information on the etiology of AKI, prognosis, pathogenesis, and treatment response.[28] SCr does not correlate with the dynamic changes in kidney function in a timely fashion and hence has a poor indicator for early diagnosis of AKI.[29] Several factors can cause a delay in the rise of SCr after the onset of AKI, such as the dilutional effect from intravenous fluids or drugs that can interfere with the tubular secretion of creatinine, to name a few.[30,31] Various serum and urinary proteins have been investigated to serve as candidate biomarkers for diagnosing AKI and localizing the site of structural damage. In addition, the National Institutes of Health (NIH)/National Institute of Diabetes and Digestive and Kidney Diseases (NIDDK) initiated the Kidney Precision Medicine Project (KPMP) in 2019; the objective of KPMP is to ethically obtain human kidney biopsy samples from participants with AKI and CKD and identify critical cells, pathways, and targets for therapy.[32] A plethora of biomarkers with varying sensitivity and specificity have been determined using proteomics as a part of KPMP.

Acute kidney injury without rise in serum creatinine
AKI can occur in the absence of a rise of SCr or a decrease in urine output, and this has led to the concept of subclinical AKI (Fig. 1, Box C). The pathophysiological explanation for this entity is that the noninjured nephrons compensate for the functional loss of the injured nephrons, also called the renal reserve. AKD is a new concept that includes AKI and the conditions associated with subacute decreases in GFR (AKD/non-

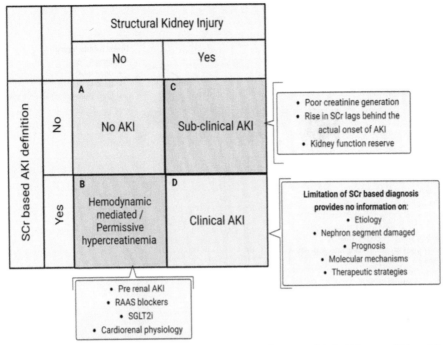

Fig. 1. A 2 × 2 grid depicting the shortcomings of SCr-based definitions of AKI. AKI, acute kidney injury; RAAS, renin-angiotensin-aldosterone system; SCr, SCr; SGLT2i, sodium-glucose transporter 2 inhibitors. (*Adapted from Moledina and colleagues*)[33]

AKI). A biopsy-proven acute tubular injury (ATI) study demonstrated that 21% of the patients did not meet the KDIGO SCr-based AKI definition.[34] The factors leading to subclinical AKI are poor creatinine generation (eg, malnutrition or poor muscle mass), the lag time (sometimes 48–72 hours) between rise of SCr and actual onset of clinical AKI and underlying kidney function reserve. Therefore, this window is clinically critical to intervene and correct the factors precipitating the AKI, e.g., nephrotoxic, or hemodynamic insult.

Rise in serum creatinine without acute kidney injury/concept of permissive hypercreatininemia

Specific processes like cardiorenal physiology, medications like renin-angiotensin and aldosterone system (RAAS) blockers, and SGLT2 inhibitors can interfere with kidney hemodynamics, leading to a rise in SCr without any demonstrable structural kidney damage (see **Fig. 1**, Box B). The most important clinical question is, *"How much acute decline in the eGFR is clinically acceptable?"* The hallmark of cardiorenal physiology is attenuated forward blood flow and venous congestion.[35] RAAS blockers, diuretics, and SGLT2 inhibitors are the pillars of managing heart failure with reduced ejection fraction

(HFrEF).[36] Both the underlying physiology and the treatment have the potential to acutely drop the GFR due to their effects on systemic and intraglomerular hemodynamics. Permissive hypercreatininemia is vital, so one does not withdraw the RAAS blockers and SGLT2 inhibitors, as a large body of evidence supports its benefit in HFrEF. Without an apparent reason for the sharp drop in GFR, the inclination should be to continue RAAS blockers for up to a 30% drop in eGFR.[37–39]

Biomarkers of acute kidney injury

The Biomarkers, EndpointS, and Other Tools (BEST) glossary define a biomarker as a characteristic that is measured as an indicator of normal biologic processes, pathogenic processes, or responses to an exposure or intervention, including therapeutic interventions (Fig. 2).[40] During the past decade, several biomarkers of AKI have been identified and investigated; however, only some biomarkers are universally available. In its quest to identify an ideal biomarker, the ADQI groups proposed a framework for using functional and damage biomarkers to stratify patients with AKI. In this narrative, we outline the existing and novel biomarkers for the diagnosis and prognosis of AKI in varied cardiological settings.[41]

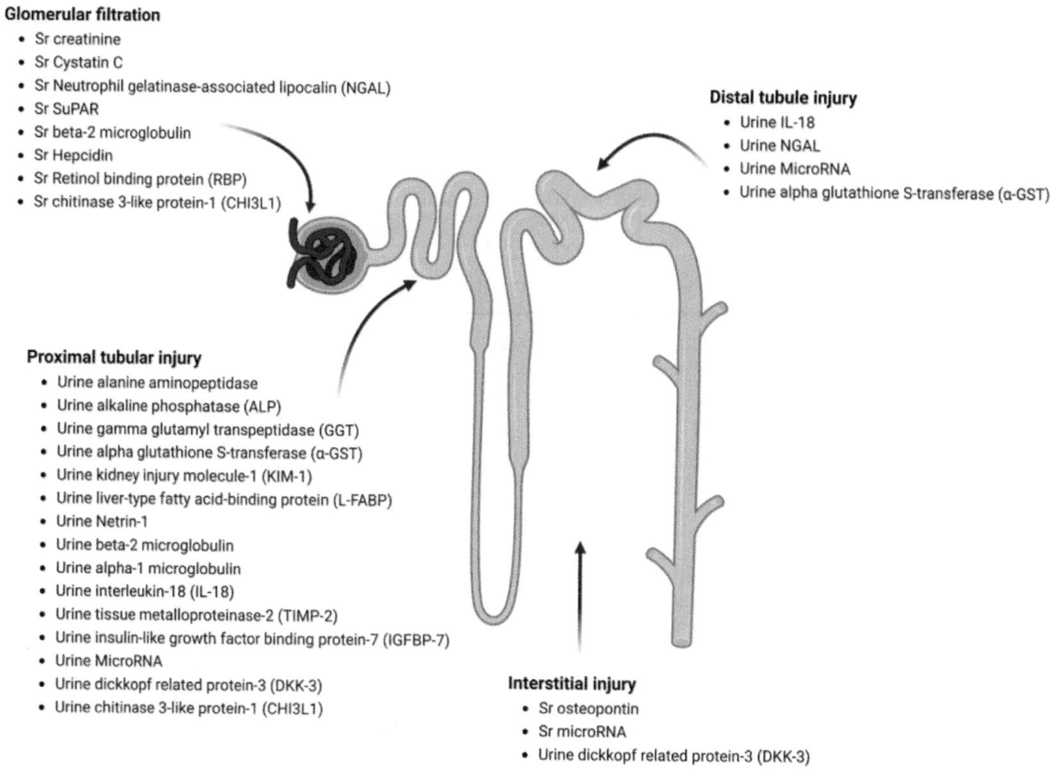

Glomerular filtration
- Sr creatinine
- Sr Cystatin C
- Sr Neutrophil gelatinase-associated lipocalin (NGAL)
- Sr SuPAR
- Sr beta-2 microglobulin
- Sr Hepcidin
- Sr Retinol binding protein (RBP)
- Sr chitinase 3-like protein-1 (CHI3L1)

Distal tubule injury
- Urine IL-18
- Urine NGAL
- Urine MicroRNA
- Urine alpha glutathione S-transferase (α-GST)

Proximal tubular injury
- Urine alanine aminopeptidase
- Urine alkaline phosphatase (ALP)
- Urine gamma glutamyl transpeptidase (GGT)
- Urine alpha glutathione S-transferase (α-GST)
- Urine kidney injury molecule-1 (KIM-1)
- Urine liver-type fatty acid-binding protein (L-FABP)
- Urine Netrin-1
- Urine beta-2 microglobulin
- Urine alpha-1 microglobulin
- Urine interleukin-18 (IL-18)
- Urine tissue metalloproteinase-2 (TIMP-2)
- Urine insulin-like growth factor binding protein-7 (IGFBP-7)
- Urine MicroRNA
- Urine dickkopf related protein-3 (DKK-3)
- Urine chitinase 3-like protein-1 (CHI3L1)

Interstitial injury
- Sr osteopontin
- Sr microRNA
- Urine dickkopf related protein-3 (DKK-3)

Fig. 2. Origin of biomarkers of AKI and its source of generation concerning nephron. IL-18, interleukin-18; Micro-RNA, micro ribose nucleic acid; Sr, serum; SuPAR, soluble urokinase plasminogen activator receptor.

Biomarkers of glomerular filtration

SCr and serum cystatin C (SrCysC) are commonly used glomerular filtration markers. SrCysC, a serine protease produced by human nucleated cells, is subject to less physical interference and is more sensitive to early declines in kidney function than SCr. It has a low molecular mass, is freely filtered by the glomeruli, and is fully catabolized in the proximal renal tubules. The combined SCr-CysC equation has been shown to outperform equations based on either marker alone for estimating GFR.[42] However, in the Translational Research Investigating Biomarker Endpoints for Acute Kidney Injury (TRIBE-AKI) Consortium cohort, SrCysC was less sensitive for AKI detection than SCr. Still, it identified a subset of patients with AKI with a substantially higher risk of adverse outcomes.[43]

Biomarkers for tubular function

Fractional excretion of sodium (FENa) and furosemide stress test (FST) are surrogate markers used to evaluate the functional integrity of tubular function. FENa may be particularly useful in patients suspected of having AKI due to prerenal disease or acute tubular necrosis (ATN). The clinical value of calculating FENa is highest in patients with oliguric AKI who have no preexisting CKD and are diuretic naive. On the other hand, FST challenges renal tubular function by administering a high dose of furosemide. Koyner and colleagues[44] found that, in the setting of early AKI, urine output measured after FST outperformed biochemical biomarkers in predicting progressive AKI, need for KRT, and inpatient mortality. Furosemide responsiveness was a better predictor of progression to AKIN stage III (area under the curve [AUC] 0.87, 95% confidence interval [CI] 0.73–0.94) and had better operating characteristics than plasma NGAL (AUC 0.80, 95% CI 0.67–0.88).[45]

Biomarkers for cardiac surgery associated acute kidney injury

Renal tubular biomarkers

Cardiac surgery-associated AKI (CSA-AKI) is a common and severe complication of cardiac surgery with a reported incidence of 5% to 42% in different settings (Table 2).[59] Timely initiation of preventive strategies, that is, "KDIGO bundle" with early detection of tubular biomarkers like tissue inhibitor of metalloproteinases 2 (TIMP-2) and insulin-like growth factor binding protein 7 (IGFBP-7) (urinary TIMP-2/IGFBP-7 > 0.3) reduces the frequency and severity of CSA-AKI.[60] A prospective observational study to assess the

Table 2
Clinical studies on utility of biomarkers for cardiac surgery associated-acute kidney injury

Sr No:	Author/Year	Type of Study and Primary Outcome	Biomarkers	AKI Early Detection	AKI Severity Prediction	Mortality Prediction	Long-Term CV/Renal Outcomes
1.	Gist et al,[46] 2017	Multicenter prospective/AKI with 72 h of surgery	uIGFBP-7*TIMP-2	Yes	Yes	-	-
2	De Loor et al,[47] 2017	Single-center prospective cohort/ AKI stage >/ = 1 within 48 h of surgery	Sr CHI3L1 + u CHIL3L1/u NGAL	Yes	Yes	-	-
3.	Coca et al,[48] 2014	Multicenter prospective cohort/ 3 y mortality	u NGAL, IL-18, KIM-1, LFABP, albumin	-	-	Yes, prediction of 3-year mortality	-
4.	Sarnak et al,[49] 2014	Prospective cohort/ all-cause mortality and CVD	u KIM-1, IL-18, albumin	-	-	Albuminuria, strongly and u KIM-1, modestly associated with all-cause mortality	Albuminuria strongly associated with CVD
5.	Parikh et al,[50] 2011	Prospective, multicenter cohort/ AKI risk prediction	u IL-18, u NGAL, Sr NGAL	Yes	Yes, AKI stage net reclassification	-	-
6.	Han et al,[51] 2009	Prospective, multicenter cohort/ AKI early detection	u KIM-1, NAG, NGAL	Yes	-	-	-
3.	Neyra et al,[52] 2019	Prospective cohort/ postop in hospital AKI	u KIM-1+ Sr CysC + clinical model	Yes	-	-	-
4.	Menez et al,[53] 2021	Prospective cohort – TRIBE-AKI/ composite of CKD incidence/ progression	Sr bFGF, Sr KIM-1, Sr NT-Pro-BNP, Sr sTNFR1	-	-	-	Independently associated with increased risk of CKD, irrespective

(continued on next page)

Table 2
(continued)

Sr No:	Author/Year	Type of Study and Primary Outcome	Biomarkers	AKI Early Detection	AKI Severity Prediction	Mortality Prediction	Long-Term CV/Renal Outcomes
							of the stage of index AKI event
5.	Cui et al,[54] 2021	Prospective cohort/AKI diagnosis	Plasma metabolites: gluconic acid, fumaric acid. pseudo uridine	Yes	-	-	-
6.	Vasquez-Rios et al,[55] 2022	Prospective cohort – TRIBE-AKI/postop long-term CV/CKD outcomes and death	Sr sTNFr1 + Sr sTNFR2 + Sr KIM-1	-	-	Yes	Yes, independently associated with an increased risk of CV events and CKD
7.	Chen et al,[56] 2020	Prospective cohort/occurrence and severity of AKI	IFN-γ, SCGF-β	Yes	Yes	Yes (secondary outcomes)	-
8.	Schunk et al,[57] 2019	Observational cohort/early AKI detection and subsequent loss of GFR	u dickkopf-3/creatinine	Yes	Yes, improved reclassification of AKI	-	Yes, independently associated with CKD at a median follow-up of 820 d
10.	Kalisnik et al,[58] 2022	Prospective cohort study/early detection of CSA-AKI	Sr CysC, SCr, Sr NGAL	Yes	-	-	-

AKI, acute kidney injury; bFGF, basic fibroblast growth factor; CKD, chronic kidney disease; CSA-AKI, cardiac surgery associated-AKI; CV, cardiovascular; CVD, cardiovascular disease; CysC, cystatin C; dickkopf-3, Dickkopf-related protein 3; GFR, glomerular filtration rate; IFN-γ, interferon-gamma; IGFBP-7, insulin like growth factor binding protein-7; IL-18, interleukin-18; KIM-1, kidney injury molecule-1; NAG, urinary N-acetyl-β-d-glycosaminidase; NT-Pro-BNP, N terminal pro-brain natriuretic peptide; SCGF-β, stem cell growth factor; Sr, serum; sTNFR1/R2, soluble tumor necrosis factor receptor 1/2; TIMP-2, tissue metalloproteinase-2; uCHI3L1, urine chitinase 3 like protein-1; uNGAL, urine neutrophil gelatinase associated lipocalin.

efficacy of combinations of urinary NGAL and kidney injury molecule-1 (KIM-1) demonstrated that urinary NGAL was relatively sensitive. In contrast, KIM-1 seemed to be specific to ischemic kidney injury. Combining the 2 biomarkers increased the accuracy of early detection of CSA-AKI (AUC 0.906).[61] A single-center study examined the utility of the combination of biomarkers Sr CysC (kidney function loss) and urine NGAL and KIM-1 (tubular damage) for predicting AKI post-CSA-AKI. This biomarker combination significantly improved the performance of the clinical model for predicting postoperative AKI (AUC for the clinical model alone: 0.77, 95% CI: 0.65–0.90 vs 0.83, 95% CI: 0.73–0.93 for the clinical model plus biomarker data, $P = 0.049$).[52] A multicenter prospective cohort study in infants undergoing cardiopulmonary bypass (CPB) assessed the utility of TIMP-2*IGFBP-7 urine concentration at 2, 6, 12, 24, 48, and 72 hours post-CPB initiation.[46] At 12 hours after CPB initiation, patients with a TIMP-2*IGFBP-7 concentration of greater than or equal to 0.78 had 3-fold higher odds of developing AKI than those with a less than 0.78 (95% CI 1.47–6.11, $P = 0.001$). The combination of TIMP-2 and IGFBP7 urine concentrations was granted marketing approval by the US Food and Drug Administration (FDA) in 2014. This test is not limited to AKI following cardiovascular interventions and is designed to assess the risk of moderate to severe AKI in all types of critically ill patients. Challenges include varying cutoff values, confounding comorbidities, costs, and better performance in known insult timing (eg, postcardiac surgery) compared to unclear onset (eg, sepsis).

Novel biomarkers for cardiac surgery associated acute kidney injury. Several studies have evaluated new biomarkers and combinations of existing ones to predict CSA-AKI and investigate its outcomes. Among these biomarkers is chitinase 3-like protein-1 (CHI3L1), a glycoprotein secreted by activated macrophages in an inflammatory milieu. In a single-center prospective cohort study, combining systemic CHI3L1 with either urine CHI3L1 or urine NGAL was a good predictor of AKI stage greater than 2 within 12 hours of postoperative ICU admission.[47] Using metabolomics to detect and measure metabolic changes has become a valuable tool in understanding the underlying causes of AKI and identifying potential treatment targets. Researchers can identify a molecular signature associated with CSA-AKI by analyzing plasma metabolites. In one study, metabolomic analysis of plasma samples taken within 24 hours following cardiac surgery revealed increased gluconic acid, fumaric acid, and pseudouridine levels in a patient with CSA-AKI.[54] The search for biomarkers is not limited to predicting AKI onset but also identifying individuals at risk for subsequent CKD and adverse cardiovascular outcomes. In a multicenter, prospective cohort study, the TRIBE-AKI group analyzed the preoperative concentration of plasma soluble tumor necrosis factor receptor 1 and 2 (sTNFR1 and 2) and KIM-1 to study postoperative long-term outcomes. The study found that sTNFR1, sTNFR2, N-terminal pro-brain-natriuretic peptide (NT-pro-BNP), and KIM-1 were independently associated with longitudinal outcomes, including death, cardiovascular events, and CKD events, after discharge from a cardiac surgery hospitalization in high-risk individuals.[53,55] A stress-induced renal tubular cell-derived secreted glycoprotein, called dickkopf-3, has been identified as a modulator of the Wnt/β-catenin signaling pathway, which promotes AKI progression to CKD. Dickkopf-3 is expressed early in the disease process, whereas renal tubular cell injury is still clinically silent. To investigate this further, Schunk and colleagues conducted an observational cohort study of 733 patients undergoing elective cardiac surgery. They also validated their findings using a cohort from the Remote Ischemic Preconditioning (RenalRIP) trial.[57] Urinary concentrations of dickkopf-3/creatinine greater than 471 pg/mg were associated with a significantly increased risk of AKI in the derivation cohort. Moreover, high urine concentrations of dickkopf-3/creatinine were independently associated with lower kidney function after a median follow-up of 820 days. These findings suggest that dickkopf-3 could be a promising biomarker for personalized precision medicine searching for AKI biomarkers.

Biomarkers for acute kidney injury in the setting of contrast exposure

When a patient experiences AKI after receiving intravenous contrast, the condition can be classified as either contrast-associated AKI (CA-AKI) or contrast-induced AKI (CI-AKI). CA-AKI is a more general term encompassing cases where AKI occurs soon after receiving iodinated contrast, but the cause may not be directly related to the contrast material.

CI-AKI, previously known as contrast-induced nephropathy, is a type of AKI specifically caused by iodinated contrast material. The contrast agents may lead to AKI by 2 main mechanisms: direct cellular toxicity and renal hemodynamic

Table 3
Clinical studies on the utility of biomarkers for contrast-associated acute kidney injury

Sr No:	Author (Year)	Study Type/ Primary Outcome	Biomarkers	AKI Early Detection	AKI Severity Prediction	Mortality Prediction	Long-Term CV/ Renal Outcomes
1.	Nozue et al,[63] 2010	Prospective cohort/AKI detection	Sr CysC, Sr β2-MG, u L-FABP, u β2-MG, urine NAG	Yes	-	-	-
2.	Li et al,[64] 2015	Prospective cohort/AKI detection	SCr, Sr CysC, Sr β2-MG	Yes	-	-	-
3.	Ren et al,[65] 2011	Prospective cohort/AKI detection	u NAG	Yes	-	-	-
4.	Quintavalle et al,[66] 2015	Prospective cohort/AKI prediction	u NGAL, Sr NGAL	Yes	-	Yes	MAE: dialysis, nonfatal MI, CKD, and myocardial revascularization at 1 y
5.	Wang et al,[67] 2016	Meta-analysis/AKI risk prediction	u NGAL, Sr NGAL	Yes	-	-	-
6.	Akdeniz et al,[68] 2015	Prospective cohort/AKI early detection	u KIM-1	Yes	-	-	-
7.	Li et al,[69] 2015	Prospective cohort/AKI early detection	u KIM-1	Yes	-	-	-
8.	Wybraniec et al,[70] 2017	Prospective observational/ AKI early detection	u IL-18, u L-FABP, u KIM-1	Joint assay—yes	-	-	-

No.	Study	Study type/purpose	Biomarker	Validation	Predictive performance	Mortality risk	Other adverse outcomes
9.	Ling et al,[71] 2008	Prospective cohort/AKI early detection	u IL-18, u NGAL	Yes	-	-	u IL-18 a/w late adverse cardiac outcomes
10.	He et al,[72] 2014	Prospective cohort/AKI risk prediction	u IL-18	Yes	-	-	-
11.	Fujita et al,[73] 2015	Prospective cohort/long-term renal outcome	u L-FABP	-	-	-	Yes, predicting 1 y renal outcome (CKD)
12.	Nakamura et al,[74] 2006	Prospective cohort/AKI early detection	u L-FABP	Yes	-	-	-
13.	Kamijo-Ikemori et al,[75] 2015	Retrospective study/risk for CV events	u L-FABP	-	-	-	An essential indicator for risk stratification for CV events
14.	Malyszko et al,[76] 2015	Prospective cohort/AKI early detection	Sr Midkine, Sr NGAL, u NGAL, Sr CysC	-	Sr Midkine predicts early ischemic/nephrotoxic AKI	-	-
15.	Peabody et al,[77] 2022	RCT/AKI risk prediction	u L-FABP	Yes	-	-	-
16.	Ahmed M et al,[78] 2020	Prospective observational/AKI early detection	Sr Midkine	Yes	-	-	-
17.	Connolly et al,[79] 2018	Prospective observation/AKI early detection	Sr NGAL, Sr L-FABP, Sr KIM-1, Sr IL-18, u NGAL, u IL-18	-	Yes, 4 h Sr L-FABP and 6 h Sr NGAL perform best	3 times increased risk for death at 1 y	4 times increased risk for MACE at 1 y
18.	Bulent Gul et al,[80] 2008	Case-control/AKI early detection	Sr IL-18	No	-	-	-

(continued on next page)

Table 3
(continued)

Sr No:	Author (Year)	Study Type/ Primary Outcome	Biomarkers	AKI Early Detection	AKI Severity Prediction	Mortality Prediction	Long-Term CV/ Renal Outcomes
19.	Bachorzewska-Gajewska et al,[81] 2009	Prospective cohort/AKI early detection	Sr NGAL, u NGAL, u L-FABP	All biomarkers increased significantly after 4 h and remained elevated for 48 h post-PCI	-	-	-
20.	Oksuz et al,[82] 2015	Prospective cohort/AKI early detection	GGT	GGT independent predictor for CIN	-	-	-

MI, myocardial infarction; a/w, associated with; AKI, acute kidney injury; CIN, contrast-induced nephropathy; CKD, chronic kidney disease; CV, cardiovascular; CysC, cystatin C; GGT, gammy glutamyl transpeptidase; MACE, major adverse cardiac events; MAE, major adverse events; post-PCI, post-percutaneous cardiac intervention; Sr NGAL, serum neutrophil gelatinase-associated lipocalin; Sr, serum; uIL-18, urine interleukin −18; uKIM-1, urine kidney injury molecule-1; uL-FABP, urine liver type fatty acid binding protein; uNAG, urine urinary N-acetyl-β-d-glycosaminidase; uNGAL, urine neutrophil gelatinase-associated lipocalin; β2-MG, beta 2 microglobulin.

Table 4
Biomarkers for prediction of acute kidney injury in acute decompensated heart failure and cardiorenal syndrome

Sr No:	Author (year)	Study Type/ Primary Outcome	Biomarkers	AKI Early Detection	AKI Severity Prediction	Mortality Prediction	Long/Short-Term CV/Renal Outcomes
1.	Hasse et al,[86] 2009	Meta-analysis/AKI prediction	Sr and u NGAL	Yes	Yes	Yes	-
2.	Mortara et al,[87] 2013	Prospective cohort/AKI prediction	Sr NGAL	Yes	-	-	-
3.	Collins et al,[88] 2012	Prospective/WRF and 5 and 30 d outcomes	u NGAL	Yes, in univariate analysis	-	-	Increased risk of 30 d CV outcomes
4.	Sokolski et al,[89] 2017	Prospective cohort/ prediction of true WRF in AHF	u NGAL, u KIM-1, u CysC	Yes, u NGAL at baseline and u KIM-1 at day 2 are early predictors.	-	u NGAL at days 2 and 3, u CysC at day 2 predicted mortality, u KIM1 did not predict mortality	-
5	Horiyuchi et al,[90] 2021	Retrospective/ prediction of WRF	Sr NGAL and u NGAL	Biomarkers are not able to predict WRF better than SCr	-	-	AKI biomarkers may predict WRF for HF hospitalizations at 1 y
6.	Murray et al,[91] 2019	Multicenter prospective/AKI early prediction or RRT initiation	u NGAL	u NGAL not superior to SCr	-	-	-
7.	Dankova et al,[92] 2020	Prospective cohort/AKI risk prediction	u NGAL, TIMP2, IGFBP7	Admission biomarkers predict AKI	-	-	-

(continued on next page)

Table 4
(continued)

Sr No:	Author (year)	Study Type/Primary Outcome	Biomarkers	AKI Early Detection	AKI Severity Prediction	Mortality Prediction	Long/Short-Term CV/Renal Outcomes
8.	Chen et al,[93] 2016	Prospective multicenter/AKI progression	u AGT, u NGAL, Sr NGAL, u IL-18, u KIM-1	-	Yes, u AGT, u NGAL and u IL-18 at AKI diagnosis predict progression	Yes, u AGT, u NGAL and u IL-18 at AKI diagnosis predicts progression	-
9.	Yang et al,[94] 2015	Prospective observational multicenter cohort/prediction of AKI	u AGT	Yes, u AGT outperformed u NGAL, UACR, and clinical model	-	Yes	-
10.	Alvelos et al,[95] 2011	Prospective cohort/detection of type 1 CRS	Sr NGAL and Sr CysC	Admission Sr NGAL predicts the onset of type 1 CRS	-	-	-
11.	Verbrugge et al,[96] 2013	Prospective/prediction of AKI, persistence, of AKI and mortality	u NGAL, KIM-1 and IL-18	Modest predictors of AKI	-	u IL-18 significantly a/all-cause mortality	u IL-18 predicted the persistence of kidney impairment
12.	Atici et al,[97] 2018	Prospective/AKI prediction	u TIMP-2, ILGF-7, KIM-1, and IGFBP-7	u ILGF-7 * TIMP-2 predict AKI	-	-	-

AGT, angiotensinogen, IL-18, interleukin-18; CRS, cardiorenal syndrome; CysC, cystatin C; IGFBP-7, insulin-like growth factor binding protein-7; KIM-1, kidney injury molecule-1; NGAL, neutrophil gelatinase-associated lipocalin; SCr, SCr; Sr, serum; TIMP-2:tissue metalloproteinase-2; u, urine; UACR, urine albumin to creatinine ratio; WRF, worsening renal function.

effects. Although SCr is still commonly used to diagnose CI-AKI, several other biomarkers, including CysC, NGAL, KI-1, IL-18, and L-FABP, have been studied and show promise in detecting AKI in its subclinical phase.[62] A review of the relevant studies on the utility of these biomarkers for CI-AKI is summarized in Table 3.

Biomarkers for prediction of acute kidney injury in acute decompensated heart failure and cardiorenal syndrome

The complex bidirectional nature of heart and kidney interaction in health and disease is called cardiorenal syndrome (CRS) and can be caused by acute or chronic cardiac or kidney disease. Type 1 CRS (acute CRS) refers to acute kidney dysfunction in ADHF. This type of CRS is triggered by a critical insult that leads to reduced cardiac output, decreased kidney perfusion pressure, increased kidney vascular resistance, and, ultimately, decreased GFR.[35] Type 1 CRS occurs in about 25% of patients hospitalized for ADHF.[83] The limitations of using SCr-based AKI definitions have been highlighted earlier. In the context of type 1 CRS, the potential usefulness of kidney biomarkers has been investigated.

In patients with ADHF, SrCysC has been demonstrated to predict rehospitalization and short-term and long-term mortality strongly. Furthermore, when combined with other cardiac biomarkers, such as NT-proBNP and cardiac troponin, SrCysC offers supplementary prognostic information that can improve the accuracy of outcome prediction for these patients.[84,85] Studies have investigated various tubular biomarkers alone or in combination, and their findings have been compiled and summarized in Table 4.

SUMMARY

AKI is a known complication and risk factor for adverse outcomes with cardiovascular disease and its interventions. The evolution in defining AKI has attempted to improve accuracy and consistency in the diagnosis. However, current (readily available) biomarkers have limitations in their utility and determination in the etiology of injury. Only a few new biomarkers have been integrated into clinical practice. NGAL is available in Europe, L-type fatty acid-binding protein is covered by insurance in Japan, and urinary (TIMP-2) × (IGFBP7) is commercially available in the United States and Europe. Biomarkers use is not without challenges and include varying cutoff values, confounding comorbidities, costs,

and better performance in known insult timing (eg, postcardiac surgery) compared with unclear onset (eg, sepsis). Advancements in novel biomarkers have shown promise in determining injury etiology and predicting risk for acute and chronic disease with adverse cardiovascular outcomes. Continued improvements are needed in defining AKI with the assistance of novel biomarkers; the goal is to improve early detection, intervention, and outcomes.

CLINICS CARE POINTS

- The definition of AKI in cardiovascular interventions has evolved with criteria such as RIFLE, AKIN, and KDIGO.
- Cardiology community uses VARC AKI definitions (VARC-1, 2, 3), which are based on RIFLE, AKIN, and KDIGO adaptations, respectively, and further updates within the council for monitoring outcomes.
- AKI can occur without a rise in SCr or a decrease in urine output. Timely identification is crucial for intervention before SCr levels rise. On the contrary, certain processes and medications can raise SCr without structural kidney damage. Determining acceptable acute decline in eGFR is crucial for medication management.
- Biomarkers have been explored to overcome these limitations, providing additional information on AKI etiology, prognosis, and treatment response. However, their clinical utility in cardiological settings is still being studied.
- AKI definitions vary and biomarkers have potential but require further research before these are ready to use for practical application.

DISCLOSURE

The authors have nothing to disclose regarding this article.

REFERENCES

1. Bellomo R, Ronco C, Kellum JA, et al. Acute dialysis quality initiative w. acute renal failure - definition, outcome measures, animal models, fluid therapy and information technology needs: the second international consensus conference of the acute dialysis quality initiative (ADQI) group. Crit Care 2004; 8(4):R204–12.

2. Mehta RL, Kellum JA, Shah SV, et al. Acute kidney injury network: report of an initiative to improve outcomes in acute kidney injury. Crit Care 2007;11(2):R31.

3. Leon MB, Piazza N, Nikolsky E, et al. Standardized endpoint definitions for transcatheter aortic valve implantation clinical trials: a consensus report from the valve academic research consortium. J Am Coll Cardiol 2011;57(3):253–69.

4. Kappetein AP, Head SJ, Genereux P, et al. Updated standardized endpoint definitions for transcatheter aortic valve implantation: the Valve Academic Research Consortium-2 consensus document. J Am Coll Cardiol 2012;60(15):1438–54.

5. Varc-3 Writing C, Genereux P, Piazza N, et al. Valve academic research consortium 3: updated endpoint definitions for aortic valve clinical research. J Am Coll Cardiol 2021;77(21):2717–46.

6. Tsai TT, Patel UD, Chang TI, et al. Contemporary incidence, predictors, and outcomes of acute kidney injury in patients undergoing percutaneous coronary interventions: insights from the NCDR Cath-PCI registry. JACC Cardiovasc Interv 2014;7(1):1–9.

7. Tsai TT, Patel UD, Chang TI, et al. Validated contemporary risk model of acute kidney injury in patients undergoing percutaneous coronary interventions: insights from the National Cardiovascular Data Registry Cath-PCI registry. J Am Heart Assoc 2014;3(6):e001380.

8. Safley DM, Salisbury AC, Tsai TT, et al. Acute kidney injury following in-patient lower extremity vascular intervention: from the national cardiovascular data registry. JACC Cardiovasc Interv 2021;14(3):333–41.

9. Grossman PM, Ali SS, Aronow HD, et al. Contrast-induced nephropathy in patients undergoing endovascular peripheral vascular intervention: Incidence, risk factors, and outcomes as observed in the blue cross blue shield of michigan cardiovascular consortium. J Interv Cardiol 2017;30(3):274–80.

10. Julien HM, Stebbins A, Vemulapalli S, et al. Incidence, predictors, and outcomes of acute kidney injury in patients undergoing transcatheter aortic valve replacement: insights from the society of thoracic surgeons/american college of cardiology national cardiovascular data registry-transcatheter valve therapy registry. Circ Cardiovasc Interv 2021;14(4):e010032.

11. Prasad A, Palevsky PM, Bansal S, et al. Management of Patients With Kidney Disease in Need of Cardiovascular Catheterization: A Scientific Workshop Cosponsored by the National Kidney Foundation and the Society for Cardiovascular Angiography and Interventions. Journal of the Society for Cardiovascular Angiography & Interventions 2022;1:100445. https://doi.org/10.1016/j.jscai.2022.100445.

12. Koifman E, Segev A, Fefer P, et al. Comparison of acute kidney injury classifications in patients undergoing transcatheter aortic valve implantation:

Predictors and long-term outcomes. Catheter Cardiovasc Interv. Feb 15 2016;87(3):523-31. doi:10.1002/ccd.26138

13. Sutherland L, Hittesdorf E, Yoh N, et al. Acute kidney injury after cardiac surgery: a comparison of different definitions. Nephrology 2020;25(3):212–8.

14. Roy AK, Mc Gorrian C, Treacy C, et al. A comparison of traditional and novel definitions (RIFLE, AKIN, and KDIGO) of acute kidney injury for the prediction of outcomes in acute decompensated heart failure. Cardiorenal Med 2013;3(1):26–37.

15. Nguyen MT, Maynard SE, Kimmel PL. Misapplications of commonly used kidney equations: renal physiology in practice. Clin J Am Soc Nephrol 2009;4(3):528–34.

16. Rabito CA, Panico F, Rubin R, et al. Noninvasive, real-time monitoring of renal function during critical care. J Am Soc Nephrol 1994;4(7):1421–8.

17. Mandelbaum T, Lee J, Scott DJ, et al. Empirical relationships among oliguria, creatinine, mortality, and renal replacement therapy in the critically ill. Intensive Care Med 2013;39(3):414–9.

18. Md Ralib A, Pickering JW, Shaw GM, et al. The urine output definition of acute kidney injury is too liberal. Crit Care 2013;17(3):R112.

19. Prowle JR, Liu YL, Licari E, et al. Oliguria as predictive biomarker of acute kidney injury in critically ill patients. Crit Care 2011;15(4):R172.

20. Macedo E, Malhotra R, Claure-Del Granado R, et al. Defining urine output criterion for acute kidney injury in critically ill patients. Nephrol Dial Transplant 2011;26(2):509–15.

21. Thomas ME, Blaine C, Dawnay A, et al. The definition of acute kidney injury and its use in practice. Kidney Int 2015;87(1):62–73.

22. Perrone RD, Madias NE, Levey AS. Serum creatinine as an index of renal function: new insights into old concepts. Clin Chem 1992;38(10):1933–53.

23. Chertow GM, Burdick E, Honour M, et al. Acute kidney injury, mortality, length of stay, and costs in hospitalized patients. J Am Soc Nephrol 2005;16(11):3365–70.

24. Lassnigg A, Schmidlin D, Mouhieddine M, et al. Minimal changes of serum creatinine predict prognosis in patients after cardiothoracic surgery: a prospective cohort study. J Am Soc Nephrol 2004;15(6):1597–605.

25. Levy MM, Macias WL, Vincent JL, et al. Early changes in organ function predict eventual survival in severe sepsis. Crit Care Med 2005;33(10):2194–201.

26. Khwaja A. KDIGO clinical practice guidelines for acute kidney injury. Nephron Clin Pract 2012;120(4):c179–84.

27. Lameire NH, Levin A, Kellum JA, et al. Harmonizing acute and chronic kidney disease definition and classification: report of a kidney disease: improving global outcomes (KDIGO) consensus conference. Kidney Int 2021;100(3):516–26.

28. Waikar SS, Betensky RA, Emerson SC, et al. Imperfect gold standards for kidney injury biomarker evaluation. J Am Soc Nephrol 2012;23(1):13–21.

29. Bonventre JV. Diagnosis of acute kidney injury: from classic parameters to new biomarkers. Contrib Nephrol 2007;156:213–9.

30. Macedo E, Bouchard J, Soroko SH, et al. Fluid accumulation, recognition and staging of acute kidney injury in critically-ill patients. Crit Care 2010;14(3):R82.

31. Zhang X, Rule AD, McCulloch CE, et al. Tubular secretion of creatinine and kidney function: an observational study. BMC Nephrol 2020;21(1):108.

32. de Boer IH, Alpers CE, Azeloglu EU, et al. Rationale and design of the kidney precision medicine project. Kidney Int 2021;99(3):498–510.

33. Moledina DG, Parikh CR. Phenotyping of acute kidney injury: beyond serum creatinine. Semin Nephrol 2018;38(1):3–11.

34. Chu R, Li C, Wang S, et al. Assessment of KDIGO definitions in patients with histopathologic evidence of acute renal disease. Clin J Am Soc Nephrol 2014;9(7):1175–82.

35. Rangaswami J, Bhalla V, Blair JEA, et al. Cardiorenal syndrome: classification, pathophysiology, diagnosis, and treatment strategies: a scientific statement from the american heart association. Circulation 2019;139(16):e840–78.

36. Haydock PM, Flett AS. Management of heart failure with reduced ejection fraction. Heart 2022;108(19):1571–9.

37. McCallum W, Tighiouart H, Ku E, et al. Acute declines in estimated glomerular filtration rate on enalapril and mortality and cardiovascular outcomes in patients with heart failure with reduced ejection fraction. Kidney Int 2019;96(5):1185–94.

38. Granger CB, McMurray JJ, Yusuf S, et al. Effects of candesartan in patients with chronic heart failure and reduced left-ventricular systolic function intolerant to angiotensin-converting-enzyme inhibitors: the CHARM-Alternative trial. Lancet 2003;362(9386):772–6.

39. Group CTS. Effects of enalapril on mortality in severe congestive heart failure. Results of the cooperative north scandinavian enalapril survival study (CONSENSUS). N Engl J Med 1987;316(23):1429–35.

40. BEST (Biomarkers, EndpointS, and other Tools) Resource. 2016.FDA-NIH Biomarker Working Group.

41. Ostermann M, Zarbock A, Goldstein S, et al. Recommendations on acute kidney injury biomarkers from the acute disease quality initiative consensus conference: a consensus statement. JAMA Netw Open 2020;3(10):e2019209.

42. Inker LA, Schmid CH, Tighiouart H, et al. Estimating glomerular filtration rate from serum creatinine and cystatin C. N Engl J Med 2012;367(1):20–9.

43. Spahillari A, Parikh CR, Sint K, et al. Serum cystatin C- versus creatinine-based definitions of acute kidney injury following cardiac surgery: a prospective cohort study. Am J Kidney Dis 2012;60(6):922–9.

44. Koyner JL, Davison DL, Brasha-Mitchell E, et al. Furosemide stress test and biomarkers for the prediction of AKI severity. J Am Soc Nephrol 2015;26(8):2023–31.

45. Matsuura R, Komaru Y, Miyamoto Y, et al. Response to different furosemide doses predicts AKI progression in ICU patients with elevated plasma NGAL levels. Ann Intensive Care 2018;8(1):8.

46. Gist KM, Goldstein SL, Wrona J, et al. Kinetics of the cell cycle arrest biomarkers (TIMP-2*IGFBP-7) for prediction of acute kidney injury in infants after cardiac surgery. Pediatr Nephrol 2017;32(9):1611–9.

47. De Loor J, Herck I, Francois K, et al. Diagnosis of cardiac surgery-associated acute kidney injury: differential roles of creatinine, chitinase 3-like protein 1 and neutrophil gelatinase-associated lipocalin: a prospective cohort study. Ann Intensive Care 2017;7(1):24.

48. Coca SG, Garg AX, Thiessen-Philbrook H, et al. Urinary biomarkers of AKI and mortality 3 years after cardiac surgery. J Am Soc Nephrol 2014;25(5):1063–71.

49. Sarnak MJ, Katz R, Newman A, et al. Association of urinary injury biomarkers with mortality and cardiovascular events. J Am Soc Nephrol 2014;25(7):1545–53.

50. Parikh CR, Coca SG, Thiessen-Philbrook H, et al. Postoperative biomarkers predict acute kidney injury and poor outcomes after adult cardiac surgery. J Am Soc Nephrol 2011;22(9):1748–57.

51. Han WK, Wagener G, Zhu Y, et al. Urinary biomarkers in the early detection of acute kidney injury after cardiac surgery. Clin J Am Soc Nephrol 2009;4(5):873–82.

52. Neyra JA, Hu MC, Minhajuddin A, et al. Kidney tubular damage and functional biomarkers in acute kidney injury following cardiac surgery. Kidney Int Rep 2019;4(8):1131–42.

53. Menez S, Moledina DG, Garg AX, et al. Results from the TRIBE-AKI Study found associations between post-operative blood biomarkers and risk of chronic kidney disease after cardiac surgery. Kidney Int 2021;99(3):716–24.

54. Cui H, Shu S, Li Y, et al. Plasma metabolites-based prediction in cardiac surgery-associated acute kidney injury. J Am Heart Assoc 2021;10(22):e021825.

55. Vasquez-Rios G, Moledina DG, Jia Y, et al. Preoperative kidney biomarkers and risks for death, cardiovascular and chronic kidney disease events after cardiac surgery: the TRIBE-AKI study. J Cardiothorac Surg 2022;17(1):338.

56. Chen Z, Hu Z, Hu Y, et al. Novel Potential Biomarker of Adult Cardiac Surgery-Associated Acute Kidney Injury. Front Physiol 2020;11:587204.

57. Schunk SJ, Zarbock A, Meersch M, et al. Association between urinary dickkopf-3, acute kidney injury, and subsequent loss of kidney function in patients undergoing cardiac surgery: an observational cohort study. Lancet 2019;394(10197):488–96.

58. Kalisnik JM, Steblovnik K, Hrovat E, et al. Enhanced detection of cardiac surgery-associated acute kidney injury by a composite biomarker panel in patients with normal preoperative kidney function. J Cardiovasc Dev Dis 2022;9(7). https://doi.org/10.3390/jcdd9070210.

59. Mehta RL, Burdmann EA, Cerda J, et al. Recognition and management of acute kidney injury in the International Society of Nephrology 0by25 Global Snapshot: a multinational cross-sectional study. Lancet 2016;387(10032):2017–25.

60. Meersch M, Schmidt C, Hoffmeier A, et al. Prevention of cardiac surgery-associated AKI by implementing the KDIGO guidelines in high risk patients identified by biomarkers: the PrevAKI randomized controlled trial. Intensive Care Med 2017;43(11):1551–61.

61. Elmedany SM, Naga SS, Elsharkawy R, et al. Novel urinary biomarkers and the early detection of acute kidney injury after open cardiac surgeries. J Crit Care 2017;40:171–7.

62. D'Amore C, Nuzzo S, Briguori C. Biomarkers of contrast-induced nephropathy:: which ones are clinically important? Interv Cardiol Clin 2020;9(3):335–44.

63. Nozue T, Michishita I, Mizuguchi I. Predictive value of serum cystatin C, beta2-microglobulin, and urinary liver-type fatty acid-binding protein on the development of contrast-induced nephropathy. Cardiovasc Interv Ther 2010;25(2):85–90.

64. Li S, Zheng Z, Tang X, et al. Preprocedure and post-procedure predictive values of serum beta2-Microglobulin for contrast-induced nephropathy in patients undergoing coronary computed tomography angiography: a comparison with creatinine-based parameters and cystatin C. J Comput Assist Tomogr 2015;39(6):969–74.

65. Ren L, Ji J, Fang Y, et al. Assessment of urinary N-acetyl-beta-glucosaminidase as an early marker of contrast-induced nephropathy. J Int Med Res 2011;39(2):647–53.

66. Quintavalle C, Anselmi CV, De Micco F, et al. Neutrophil gelatinase-associated lipocalin and contrast-induced acute kidney injury. Circ Cardiovasc Interv 2015;8(9):e002673.

67. Wang K, Duan CY, Wu J, et al. Predictive value of neutrophil gelatinase-associated lipocalin for contrast-induced acute kidney injury after cardiac catheterization: a meta-analysis. Can J Cardiol 2016;32(8):1033 e19–e29.

68. Akdeniz D, Celik HT, Kazanci F, et al. Is kidney injury molecule 1 a valuable tool for the early diagnosis of contrast-induced nephropathy? J Investig Med 2015;63(8):930–4.

69. Li W, Yu Y, He H, et al. Urinary kidney injury molecule-1 as an early indicator to predict contrast-induced acute kidney injury in patients with diabetes mellitus undergoing percutaneous coronary intervention. Biomed Rep 2015;3(4):509–12.

70. Wybraniec MT, Chudek J, Bozentowicz-Wikarek M, et al. Prediction of contrast-induced acute kidney injury by early post-procedural analysis of urinary biomarkers and intra-renal Doppler flow indices in patients undergoing coronary angiography. J Interv Cardiol 2017;30(5):465–72.

71. Ling W, Zhaohui N, Ben H, et al. Urinary IL-18 and NGAL as early predictive biomarkers in contrast-induced nephropathy after coronary angiography. Nephron Clin Pract 2008;108(3):c176–81.

72. He H, Li W, Qian W, et al. Urinary interleukin-18 as an early indicator to predict contrast-induced nephropathy in patients undergoing percutaneous coronary intervention. Exp Ther Med 2014;8(4):1263–6.

73. Fujita D, Takahashi M, Doi K, et al. Response of urinary liver-type fatty acid-binding protein to contrast media administration has a potential to predict one-year renal outcome in patients with ischemic heart disease. Heart Ves 2015;30(3):296–303.

74. Nakamura T, Sugaya T, Node K, et al. Urinary excretion of liver-type fatty acid-binding protein in contrast medium-induced nephropathy. Am J Kidney Dis 2006;47(3):439–44.

75. Kamijo-Ikemori A, Hashimoto N, Sugaya T, et al. Elevation of urinary liver-type fatty acid binding protein after cardiac catheterization related to cardiovascular events. Int J Nephrol Renovascular Dis 2015;8:91–9.

76. Malyszko J, Bachorzewska-Gajewska H, Koc-Zorawska E, et al. Midkine: a novel and early biomarker of contrast-induced acute kidney injury in patients undergoing percutaneous coronary interventions. BioMed Res Int 2015;2015:879509.

77. Peabody J, Paculdo D, Valdenor C, et al. Clinical utility of a biomarker to detect contrast-induced acute kidney injury during percutaneous cardiovascular procedures. Cardiorenal Med 2022;12(1):11–9.

78. Ahmed M, Abdelnabi M, Almaghraby A, et al. CRT-100.94 midkine as an early predictor of contrast-induced acute kidney injury. J Am Coll Cardiol Intv 2020;13(4 Supplement S):S26.

79. Connolly M, Kinnin M, McEneaney D, et al. Prediction of contrast induced acute kidney injury using novel biomarkers following contrast coronary angiography. QJM 2018;111(2):103–10.

80. Bulent Gul CB, Gullulu M, Oral B, et al. Urinary IL-18: a marker of contrast-induced nephropathy following percutaneous coronary intervention? Clin Biochem 2008;41(7–8):544–7.

81. Bachorzewska-Gajewska H, Poniatowski B, Dobrzycki S. NGAL (neutrophil gelatinase-associated lipocalin) and L-FABP after percutaneous coronary interventions due to unstable angina in patients with normal serum creatinine. Adv Med Sci 2009;54(2):221–4.

82. Oksuz F, Yarlioglues M, Cay S, et al. Predictive value of gamma-glutamyl transferase levels for contrast-induced nephropathy in patients with ST-segment elevation myocardial infarction who underwent primary percutaneous coronary intervention. Am J Cardiol 2015;116(5):711–6.

83. Dar O, Cowie MR. Acute heart failure in the intensive care unit: epidemiology. Crit Care Med 2008; 36(1 Suppl):S3–8.

84. Lassus J, Harjola VP, Sund R, et al. Prognostic value of cystatin C in acute heart failure in relation to other markers of renal function and NT-proBNP. Eur Heart J 2007;28(15):1841–7.

85. Manzano-Fernandez S, Boronat-Garcia M, Albaladejo-Oton MD, et al. Complementary prognostic value of cystatin C, N-terminal pro-B-type natriuretic Peptide and cardiac troponin T in patients with acute heart failure. Am J Cardiol 2009; 103(12):1753–9.

86. Haase M, Bellomo R, Devarajan P, et al. Accuracy of neutrophil gelatinase-associated lipocalin (NGAL) in diagnosis and prognosis in acute kidney injury: a systematic review and meta-analysis. Am J Kidney Dis 2009;54(6):1012–24.

87. Mortara A, Bonadies M, Mazzetti S, et al. Neutrophil gelatinase-associated lipocalin predicts worsening of renal function in acute heart failure: methodological and clinical issues. J Cardiovasc Med 2013;14(9):629–34.

88. Collins SP, Hart KW, Lindsell CJ, et al. Elevated urinary neutrophil gelatinase-associated lipocalcin after acute heart failure treatment is associated with worsening renal function and adverse events. Eur J Heart Fail 2012;14(9):1020–9.

89. Sokolski M, Zymlinski R, Biegus J, et al. Urinary levels of novel kidney biomarkers and risk of true worsening renal function and mortality in patients with acute heart failure. Eur J Heart Fail 2017; 19(6):760–7.

90. Horiuchi YU, Wettersten N, Veldhuisen DJV, et al. Potential utility of cardiorenal biomarkers for prediction and prognostication of worsening renal function in acute heart failure. J Card Fail 2021; 27(5):533–41.

91. Murray PT, Wettersten N, van Veldhuisen DJ, et al. Utility of urine neutrophil gelatinase-associated lipocalin for worsening renal function during hospitalization for acute heart failure: primary findings of the urine n-gal acute kidney injury n-gal evaluation of symptomatic heart failure study (AKINESIS). J Card Fail 2019;25(8):654–65.

92. Dankova M, Minarikova Z, Danko J, et al. Novel biomarkers for prediction of acute kidney injury in acute heart failure. Bratisl Lek Listy 2020;121(5):321–4.

93. Chen C, Yang X, Lei Y, et al. Urinary biomarkers at the time of AKI diagnosis as predictors of progression of AKI among patients with acute cardiorenal syndrome. Clin J Am Soc Nephrol 2016;11(9): 1536–44.

94. Yang X, Chen C, Tian J, et al. Urinary angiotensinogen level predicts AKI in acute decompensated heart failure: a prospective, two-stage study. J Am Soc Nephrol 2015;26(8):2032–41.

95. Alvelos M, Pimentel R, Pinho E, et al. Neutrophil gelatinase-associated lipocalin in the diagnosis of type 1 cardio-renal syndrome in the general ward. Clin J Am Soc Nephrol 2011;6(3):476–81.

96. Verbrugge FH, Dupont M, Shao Z, et al. Novel urinary biomarkers in detecting acute kidney injury, persistent renal impairment, and all-cause mortality following decongestive therapy in acute decompensated heart failure. J Card Fail 2013;19(9): 621–8.

97. Atici A, Emet S, Cakmak R, et al. Type I cardiorenal syndrome in patients with acutely decompensated heart failure: the importance of new renal biomarkers. Eur Rev Med Pharmacol Sci 2018;22(11): 3534–43.

Contrast-Associated Acute Kidney Injury
Definitions, Epidemiology, Pathophysiology, and Implications

Lalith Vemireddy, MD[a,*], Shweta Bansal, MD[b]

KEYWORDS

- Contrast-associated acute kidney injury • Definitions • Pathophysiology and outcomes

KEY POINTS

- Because, in most scenarios, it is not possible to establish causality despite extensive clinical evaluation, contrast-associated AKI (CA-AKI) has become a widely accepted term to define AKI postcontrast exposure.
- CA-AKI is diagnosed with an increase in serum creatinine by more than or equal to 0.3 mg/dL within 48 hours or greater than or equal to 50% within 7 days after contrast administration.
- True incidence of CA-AKI is hard to assess, but in the contemporary analyses, it has been reported to occur in about 7% to 9% patients, with less than 1% patients requiring dialysis.
- Hemodynamic changes, direct tubular injury, and formation of reactive oxygen species/free radicals are the proposed mechanisms involved in AKI after administration of contrast media.
- CA-AKI has been associated with worse clinical outcomes including chronic kidney disease progression, cardiovascular events, and mortality; however, discussions are ongoing regarding whether CA-AKI is a marker of an increased risk of adverse outcomes or a mediator of such outcomes.

INTRODUCTION

Iodinated contrast material is the most commonly prescribed agent in the current practice. Approximately more than 30 million doses are administered per year.[1] Acute kidney injury (AKI) is a common occurrence after intra-arterial or intravenous administration of contrast media (CM). Many terminologies and criteria have been suggested and used to define AKI, which can be either causally linked or just associated with contrast administration. Most of the understanding and pathophysiology of AKI postcontrast in human kidney is speculated from the studies on animals and uncontrolled human studies.[2] Hemodynamic changes, direct tubular injury due to formation of reactive oxygen species/free radicals, and osmotic stress are the proposed mechanisms involved in AKI after administration of CM.[2] In this article, we aim to define AKI postcontrast administration and describe its epidemiology, pathogenesis, and potential implications to patients and clinicians.

DEFINITIONS

AKI that occurs after administration of contrast material has historically been called contrast-induced nephropathy or contrast-induced AKI (CI-AKI). This entity was first described in a

a Division of Nephrology, Department of Medicine, The University of Texas Health at San Antonio, 7703 Floyd Curl Drive, MSC 7882, San Antonio, TX 78229, USA; b Division of Nephrology, The University of Texas Health at San Antonio, San Antonio, TX, USA
* Corresponding author.
E-mail address: vemireddy@uthscsa.edu
Twitter: @reddy_lalith (L.V.); @SBansalNeph (S.B.)

Intervent Cardiol Clin 12 (2023) 489–498
https://doi.org/10.1016/j.iccl.2023.06.007
2211-7458/23/© 2023 Elsevier Inc. All rights reserved.

patient who had iodinated contrast administration for intravenous pyelography to evaluate the cause for mildly elevated blood urea nitrogen and look for urinary stone and obstruction; he developed anuria in 48 hours. However, now it has been learnt that AKI may or may not be directly caused by the contrast material. Patients who require the administration of contrast usually have many other risk factors for the development of AKI that may cause or contribute to the AKI at the same time as the contrast administration, hence the proposal of use of term contrast-associated AKI (CA-AKI) instead of CI-AKI. CI-AKI can be used for the subset of AKI that is judged to be causally linked to contrast administration. However, because, in most scenarios, it is not possible to establish causality despite extensive clinical evaluation, CA-AKI has become a widely accepted and used term to define AKI postcontrast administration.

Criteria to define AKI has been an evolving process over the past 2 decades. In 2004, the Acute Dialysis Quality Initiative group published the first landmark consensus definition of AKI in adults—the Risk, Injury, Failure, Loss, and End-stage renal disease (RIFLE) classification in 5 stages.[3] Recognizing the limitation of RIFLE classification, AKI Network (AKIN) published their AKI classification for adults in 2007, an evolution of the RIFLE criteria.[4] The International Kidney Disease Improving Global Outcomes (KDIGOs) guideline merged RIFLE and AKIN to improve sensitivity and specificity in 2012.[5] AKI definitions have evolved in the same fashion in cardiovascular (CV) literature. CA-AKI has most commonly been defined in the CV literature as an increase in serum or plasma creatinine (SCr) levels by greater than or equal to 25% or greater than or equal to 0.5 mg/dL at 48 to 72 hours[6]; however, an increase in SCr has been seen starting as late as fifth day postcontrast administration, hence the adoption to latest KDIGO criteria that define CA-AKI as an increase in SCr by greater than or equal to 0.3 mg/dL within 48 hours or greater than or equal to 50% within 7 days after contrast administration. The Valve Academic Research Consortium (VARC) developed AKI definition to monitor complications after heart valve procedures, and VARC has also adopted and evolved along with RIFLE, AKIN, and KDIGO criteria. The latest VARC-3 adopts KDIGO criteria except excluding urine output due to its challenges in the clinical practice and separating the need for renal replacement therapy (RRT) as stage IV AKI.[7] Given the wide acceptance and external validation, it is recommended to use KDIGO/VARC-3 criteria to define CA-AKI.

EPIDEMIOLOGY OF CONTRAST-ASSOCIATED ACUTE KIDNEY INJURY

The true incidence rate of CA-AKI is hard to assess due to wide variation in the reported rates depending on the definitions of AKI used and patient population studied with different baseline risk factors. The rate as low as less than 1% has been reported in patient population with no risk factors and as high as greater than 20% in patients with multiple risk factors, reemphasizing the importance of use of term CA-AKI.[8] In the estimates based on large National Cardiovascular Data Registry (NCDR) Cath-percutaneous coronary intervention (PCI) database including 985,737 patients undergoing elective and urgent PCI from June 2009 through June 2011, the incidence of CA-AKI was 7.1%; dialysis was required in 0.3% of cases.[9] A latest meta-analysis by Wu and colleagues[10] demonstrated an incidence rate of CA-AKI in 9% and need for RRT in 0.5% patients receiving angiography. This study also confirmed the findings of study by Schonenberger and colleagues[11] showing higher risk of CA-AKI with intra-arterial administration compared with intravenous.

PATHOPHYSIOLOGY OF CONTRAST-ASSOCIATED ACUTE KIDNEY INJURY

The pathophysiology of CA-AKI is complex and not very well understood. Most of the understanding comes from animal models, ex vivo human vessels, uncontrolled human studies, and anecdotal observations. It is important to know that in these preclinical models, much higher doses of CM were used compared with what is typically used for diagnostic and interventional studies in humans.[12] Three important pathways have been proposed in the pathophysiology of CA-AKI and these are potentially interactive[2,6] and are discussed later.

Direct Tubular Cell Injury and Toxicity
CM are benzene derivatives that are triiodinated, and the iodine component gives the radio-opaque nature of CM.[13] It has been long established that the free, noncomplexed iodine (I2) and water polarized iodine form (H_2OI^+) are important in the microbicidal action of iodine.[14] This action is achieved by iodine reacting with several amino acids of the bacterial cell membrane proteins, which leads to loss of integrity of the cell membrane, eventually leading to

cell death.[15] Earlier versions of CM were thought to cause injury due to their high osmolarity and ionic strength. The higher osmolarity and viscosity can change the tubular flow rates that could result in local ischemia by enhancing the energy requirements to reabsorb this high osmolar load. This phenomenon leads to swelling and vacuolization of the renal proximal tubular cells, causing what is described as osmotic nephrosis[16,17] (**Fig. 1**). The newer low-osmolar (still higher osmolality than plasma) and iso-osmolar CM, despite having a lower osmolarity compared with initial CM, have still been shown to have a direct effect on human cells, especially the renal tubular epithelial cells and endothelial cells.[13]

These CM also contain at least 1 carboxyl group and is shown to be chemotoxic.[14] CM has been proposed to activate several signaling pathways involved in the apoptosis of the cells through activation of BCL-2, caspase-3, and caspase-9 leading to DNA fragmentation, altered mitochondrial function, intercellular junction damage, and loss of cell membrane protein integrity.[13,18,19] Liu and colleagues[20] also proposed that CM induced overexpression of microRNA-188 regulates SRSF7 gene, which further induces apoptosis and is a potential target for future therapies. All these pathways eventually lead to tubular damage, cast formation, and obstruction of tubular flow, increasing the intratubular pressure.

Oxidative Stress and Hypoxia

Physiologically, oxygen-free radicles and reactive oxygen species (ROS) play a critical role in regulating tubular transport, especially in medullary thick ascending limb of loop of Henle.[21,22] Oxygen-free radicals are molecules that contain one or more unpaired electrons, such as superoxide (O_2^-) and hydroxyl radical (OH^-), and these are generated by the nicotinamide adenine dinucleotide phosphate-oxidase present in the mitochondria. Less aggressively reacting molecules, such as hydrogen peroxide ($H_2O_{2)}$, are called ROS. The medullary area has abundant mitochondria and serves as a major source of ROS and free radical formation.[21] These ROS and free radicals participate in cellular signaling pathways including control of release of calcium and modulation of messengers and transcription factors such as tyrosine kinases, nuclear factor-kB, and hypoxia inducible factor.[23–25] ROS also play a role in regulating tubular microcirculation

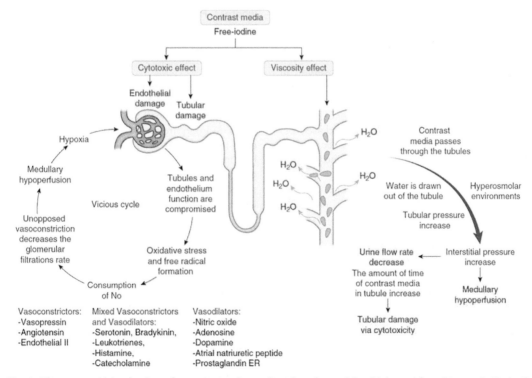

Fig. 1. The proposed mechanism of contrast-media-mediated nephrotoxicity. (*Adapted from* Morcos R, Kucharik M, Bansal P, et al. Contrast-induced acute kidney injury: review and practical update. Clinical Medicine Insights: Cardiology Volume 13: 1–9; with permission.)

through modifying nitric oxide (NO) levels.[26] However, these ROS and free radicals can become detrimental in pathological circumstances when the production increases.

CM through their strong oxidizing power stimulates the synthesis of oxygen-free radicals and ROS. Oxygen-free radicals are usually turned into water during successive reduction reaction,[2,27] but there can be an imbalance between oxidants and antioxidants with CM administration favoring oxidants. This imbalance can affect nuclear DNA, membrane/cellular lipids and proteins, as well as mitochondrial activity. ROS also activates N-terminal kinases, P38 mitogen-activated protein kinases, and stress kinases, leading to apoptosis and necrosis.[28] Furthermore, ROS and free radicals induce an increase in the synthesis of endothelin, angiotensin II, adenosine, and thromboxane A2 and a reduction in the synthesis of vasodilative NO.[26,29] As a result, the vasa recta, peritubular capillaries, and glomerular capillaries acquire a "vasoconstriction" phenotype causing alteration of renal microcirculation, reducing medullary blood flow, distal ischemia, and hypoxia. Ischemia and hypoxia further enhance the production of ROS and free radicals setting up a vicious cycle (see Fig. 1).

In anesthetized dogs, reduction in medullary flow associated with reduction in renal blood flow post-CM administration has shown to increase renal venous malondialdehyde (MDA), a marker for lipid peroxidation, up to 4-fold.[30] Furthermore, similar findings were observed in hypovolemic rats with an increase in blood MDA levels and reduction in blood thiol groups. In these models, the administration of scavengers such as superoxide dismutase, and ascorbic acid or xanthine-oxidase inhibitor allopurinol, has been shown to prevent the increase in MDA and decrease in renal blood flow.[30–32] Clinical studies had comparable findings demonstrating urinary F2 isoprostane excretion (another marker of lipid peroxidation) increased in patients after coronary angiography.[33] Urinary xanthine was also noted to be increased in patients after administration of high osmolar contrast agents, potentially suggesting that there is ROS generation.[32,33]

Notably the ability to accommodate oxidative injury decreases with age.[34,35] Furthermore, patients with chronic kidney disease (CKD) and diabetes already have increased oxidative stress, vasoconstrictors, and endothelial dysfunction explaining the increased susceptibility to CA-AKI in the elderly and patients with diabetes and CKD after contrast exposure.[36] Patients with CKD had up to 3-fold increase in urinary F2 isoprostane excretion after coronary angiography.[33]

Hemodynamic Changes Postcontrast Administration

Kidney receives up to 25% of the cardiac output, and most of the flow goes to the cortex to maintain glomerular filtration rate and reabsorption of solutes and water.[37] Renal medullary blood flow accounts for only 10% of total flow to the kidneys and primarily contributes to countercurrent multiplier system to generate osmotic gradient to enable water absorption.[38] Medullary blood flow arises from the efferent arterioles of juxtamedullary glomeruli that give rise to descending vasa recta (DVR) at corticomedullary junction. The DVR then forms a capillary bed deep into the inner medulla with accompanying histologic changes. These capillaries eventually coalesce to form ascending vasa recta (AVR) (Fig. 2).[38] Reabsorption of the sodium in the metabolically active thick ascending limbs of the loop of Henle, requiring relatively large amounts of oxygen, is a crucial step to generate the osmotic gradient involving DVR and AVR.[37] Under physiologic circumstances, oxygen partial pressure (PO_2) level of the renal cortex is approximately 50 mm Hg, whereas PO_2 levels of the renal medulla can be as low as 10 mm Hg (see Fig. 2). Because of low PO_2 but high oxygen demand, the outer medullary area is very sensitive to hemodynamic changes.[37]

CM after intravenous administration gets distributed to intravascular and interstitial space with distribution half-life of about several minutes ranging from 2 to 30 minutes.[39] CM is only 1% to 3% protein bound, not metabolized in humans but rapidly gets eliminated through glomerular filtration by the kidneys. As per studies, the elimination half-life has been noted to be 1 to 2 hours. In patients with normal kidney function, almost 100% of CM is excreted in the first 24 hours; however, it is prolonged up to 40 hours in patients with reduced kidney function.[39] Alternative routes of elimination, such as biliary elimination, are slow.

Administration of intra-arterial CM leads to biphasic hemodynamic response, initially causing increased renal blood flow followed by a prolonged decline up to 25% from baseline.[2,40,41] Even though there is a predominant decline in cortical blood flow, a mild decrease in medullary blood flow results in drop of medullary PO_2 from 20 mm Hg to as low as 9 mm Hg.[27,41] The pathogenesis of reduced medullary blood flow after

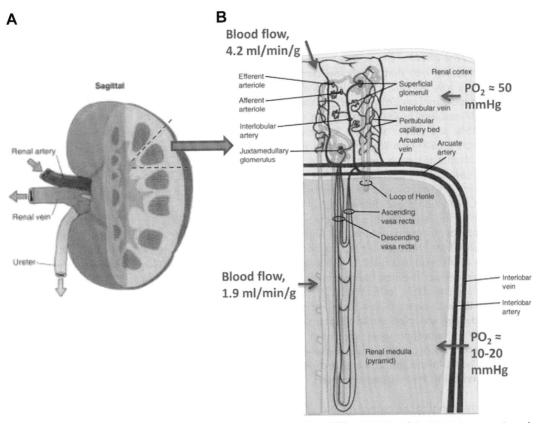

Fig. 2. (*A, B*) Anatomy of vascularization and (patho)physiology of medulla. The PO2 of the cortex is approximately 50 mm Hg and decreases to 25 mm Hg after CM administration. The PO2 of the medulla is approximately 20 mm Hg and decreases to 9 to 15 mm Hg after CM administration. The most vulnerable part for ischemia is the thick ascending limb from the loop of Henle in the outer medulla. (*From* [A] Costanzo L. Physiology. 6th ed. Elsevier; 2017, Chapter 6; [B] Boron W, Boulpaep E. Medical Physiology. 3rd ed. Elsevier; 2016, Chapter 33; with permission.)

CM has been investigated. The average diameter of DVR is about 12 to 18 μm (close to that of red blood cell, 8 μm), and on isolated rat DVR, microperfusion with iodixanol (iso-osmolar CM) causes almost 48% reduction in the diameter likely due to increased reactivity to angiotensin II. The addition of a free radical scavenger prevented this vasoconstriction induced by iodixanol and angiotensin II, suggesting direct role of oxidative stress.[42] Moreover, perfusion of human and rat renal arteries (interlobar) with CM has been shown to cause endothelial cell damage, leading to increased endothelial permeability and decreased NO availability. The pretreatment of animals with phosphodiesterase type 5 inhibitor or nitrite infusion that increase NO availability was associated with lesser degree of histological injury and attenuation in markers of AKI.[12,43] Based on these experiments, it has been postulated that DVR constriction is a consequence of oxidative stress, endothelial damage, and decreased NO availability.[29]

Prominent medullary vasodilators include adenosine, dopamine, NO, atrial natriuretic peptide, and prostaglandin E2.[37,40] Potent vasoconstrictors include vasopressin, angiotensin II, and endothelin.[37,41] Potential additional participants, with both dilative and constrictive properties, are serotonin, bradykinin, leukotrienes, histamine, and catecholamines.[40] Overall, after contrast exposure, release of adenosine, endothelin, and renin-angiotensin-aldosterone system mediators leads to afferent arteriolar vasoconstriction. On the other hand, a decline in NO and prostacyclin results in efferent arteriolar constriction. These imbalances between vasoconstrictive and vasodilation mediators in favor of the vasoconstrictive mediators lead to lower flow in peritubular capillaries and potential ischemic changes, particularly in the tubules located in watershed areas, and promote direct cell toxicity as a result of hypoxia[44] (see Fig. 1).

Of note, all these experiments have been conducted with iodixanol (iso-osmolar) as the agent investigated; it would be interesting to repeat these experiments with low-osmolar CM. The only study evaluating CM with different osmolarity compared the effect of the high-osmolar ionic CM amidotrizoate with that of the low-osmolar ioxaglate, the low-osmolar iopromide, and the iso-osmolar iodixanol on DVR constriction. All 4 types of CM resulted in DVR constriction rates between 45% and 63%, and the differences were not statistically significant.[45] Many other risks and advantages have been theorized for iso- versus low-contrast CM; however, in clinical studies, there are not any differences in incidences of CI-AKI with these different CM.[46]

With advancing age, there is a decrease in renal plasma flow as well as glomerular filtration rate and a significant reduction in Kf (capillary ultrafiltration coefficient) as a result of reduction in both the glomerular capillary permeability and the surface area available for filtration.[47,48] Similarly, patients with heart failure have reduced renal blood flow and glomerular filtration rate as a result of neurohormonal activation and inflammation.[49] As a consequence, elderly patients with heart failure are at increased risk of CI-AKI, given their already compromised renal blood flow.

After understanding the pathophysiology, it is intuitive why factors such as age, presence of diabetes, CKD, heart failure, and hypotension are associated with high risk of developing AKI after contrast exposure. These comorbidities are associated with altered hemodynamics, increased inflammation, and oxidative stress exhausting the renal reserve already, thus making one prone for increase in creatinine with any additional insults.

IMPLICATIONS OF CONTRAST-ASSOCIATED ACUTE KIDNEY INJURY

CA-AKI have been associated with not only short- and long-term clinical adverse effects such as CKD progression, cardiovascular events, and mortality but also economic implications. In the NCDR Cath-PCI registry, the in-hospital mortality rate was 9.7% for patients with CA-AKI (based on AKIN criteria) and 34% for those requiring dialysis compared with 0.5% for patients without AKI (p < 0.001). After multivariable adjustment, CA-AKI (odd ratio [OR]: 7.8; 95% confidence interval [CI]: 7.4–8.1, p < 0.001) and dialysis (OR: 21.7; 95%CI: 19.6–24.1; p < 0.001) remained independent predictors of in-hospital mortality.[50] One contemporary study evaluated 2-year mortality in the ADAPT-DES (Assessment of Dual Antiplatelet

Therapy with Drug-Eluting Stents) registry of 8582 patients treated with more than or equal to 1 drug-eluting stent. CA-AKI was defined as a post-PCI increase in SCr of greater than 0.5 mg/dL or greater than or equal to 25% and occurred in 6.5% of patients.[51] Two-year mortality was higher in patients with CA-AKI (hazard ratio [HR]: 1.77; 95% CI: 1.22–2.55) as compared with non-CA-AKI patients. The mortality rate in the contemporary analyses are somewhat better than previously reported by Gruberg and colleagues and McCullough and colleagues in early 2000s[52,53]; however, they still remain significantly higher.

In both NCRD-Cath PCI and ADAPT-DES, both short-term and long-term rates of major bleeding (OR: 2.38; 95% CI: 2.27–2.49 and HR: 1.38; 95% CI: 1.06–1.80, respectively), in-stent thrombosis/myocardial infarction rates (OR: 1.66; 95%CI: 1.58–1.75 and HR: 1.71; 95%CI: 1.10–2.65, respectively) were higher in patients with CA-AKI despite the adjustment of all the confounding risk variables.[50,51] Patients with AKI needing dialysis had an even higher rates of these complications. In earlier reports, the rates of major adverse cardiovascular events (MACE), both in-hospital and at 1 year, were higher in patients with CA-AKI regardless of presence of underlying CKD and periprocedural hemodynamic parameters.[54] CA-AKI was also associated with the progression of CKD. A study including 531 patients with acute coronary syndrome undergoing PCI reported that CA-AKI was an independent predictor for the development of sustained reduction in renal function at 6 to 8 months (40% in patients with CA-AKI vs 11% in the control group).[55]

Aubry and colleagues analyzed the French hospital discharge database including almost 1 million hospitalizations to assess the economic impact. CA-AKI was suspected in 3.1% and RRT was required in 0.6% hospitalized patients. The mean length of stay and cost of hospitalizations associated with suspected CA-AKI was higher than in hospitalizations without suspected CA-AKI (20.5 vs 4.7 days, p < 0.00001 and €15,765 vs €3,352, p < 0.0001, respectively).[56] Another study developed a decision analytical model using the model parameters obtained from the literature review to estimate the in-hospital as well as 1-year costs of CA-AKI using several databases including Medline and the Cochrane Library. The average in-hospital cost of CA-AKI was $10,345 (range $5032–12,959), and the 1-year follow-up cost was $1467 ($422 due to dialysis and $1045 related to MACE). The largest cost driver was the increased length of stay associated with the initial hospitalization. The cost estimates were almost 6 to 7 times higher in high-risk group compared with low-risk group for CA-AKI.[57] Of note, all these economic reports have not considered indirect costs due to loss of work and several other factors; therefore, the actual economic burden could be much higher than what is estimated.

This section cannot be completed without discussing the concern of residual confounding in all of these single-arm uncontrolled prospective studies that report CA-AKI as an independent predictor of worse outcomes. In a study using propensity score–matched analysis in a cohort of 21,346 patients undergoing computed tomography (10,673 in the contrast group, 10,673 in the noncontrast group), the risks of AKI (OR, 0.94; 95%CI: 0.83–1.07), emergent dialysis (OR, 0.96;95%CI: 0.54–1.60), and 30-day mortality (HR: 0.97; 95% CI: 0.87–1.06) were not significantly different between the contrast group and the noncontrast group.[58] Many more recent studies using same approach have suggested that incidence of CA-AKI is overestimated.[59–61] Moreover, the fluctuation in SCr meeting criteria of stage I AKI in hospitalized patients without contrast exposure occurs commonly, and most of the CA-AKI cases sustain stage I AKI, thus suggesting overestimation of CA-AKI incidence in patients exposed to contrast.[62] A discussion is in place regarding whether CA-AKI is a marker of an increased risk of adverse outcomes or a mediator of such outcomes. Interestingly, in a post hoc exploratory mediation analysis of 4418 participants in the PRESERVE (Prevention of Serious Adverse Outcomes Following Angiography) trial, CA-AKI was associated with an increased relative risk for 90-day death, need for dialysis, or persistent kidney impairment (OR: 3.93; 95% CI: 2.82–5.49); however, it did not mediate the association of the preangiography kidney function with these outcomes. This topic is discussed in more detail in Radha K. Adusumilli and Steven Coca's article, "Renalism: Avoiding Procedure, More Harm Than Good?" in this issue.

SUMMARY

Because, in most scenarios, it is not possible to establish causality despite extensive clinical evaluation, CA-AKI has become a widely accepted term to define AKI postcontrast, and KDIGO 2012 AKI definition is recommended to diagnose CA-AKI. Although there is clear evidence of potential nephrotoxic mechanisms in animal models including vasoconstriction, the formation of reactive oxygen species, and direct tubular toxicity, their physiologic relevance in humans is controversial. Nonetheless, based on these mechanisms, it is intuitive why the preexistent risk factors such as advance age, heart failure, chronic kidney disease, and diabetes, which cause decreased renal blood flow, altered vasoactive mediators, and increased oxidative stress, further compound these pathophysiologic mechanisms and make these patients very susceptible to CA-AKI. The 2 types of frequently used CM—low-osmolar and iso-osmolar—have their theoretic advantages and disadvantages related to their hyperosmolarity and hyperviscocity, respectively, relative to blood; however, clinically the difference in incidence of CI-AKI has not been evident. CA-AKI is associated with worse clinical outcomes such as mortality, CKD progression, and cardiovascular events; however, discussions are ongoing whether CA-AKI is a marker of an increased risk of adverse outcomes or a mediator of such outcomes.

CLINICS CARE POINTS

- Acute kidney injury (AKI) is a common occurrence after contrast media administration.

- Hemodynamic changes, direct tubular injury, and reactive oxygen species are the proposed mechanisms involved in AKI.

- Patients who require the administration of contrast usually have many other risk factors for the development of AKI and one must remain vigilant for these other risk factors instead of attributing any rise in creatinine after contrast administration to contrast itself. For the same reason, contrast- associated AKI has been the preferred term over contrast-induced AKI in these scenarios.

- KDIGO criteria are the most acceptable criteria and define CA-AKI as an increase in serum creatinine by greater than or equal to 0.3 mg/dL within 48 hours or greater than or equal to 50% within 7 days after contrast administration.

DISCLAIMER

The authors have nothing to disclose.

REFERENCES

1. Solomon R. Contrast media: are there differences in nephrotoxicity among contrast media? BioMed Res Int 2014;2014:934947.

2. Katzberg RW. Contrast medium-induced nephrotoxicity: which pathway? Radiology 2005;235(3):752–5.

3. Bellomo R, Ronco C, Kellum JA, et al. Acute dialysis quality initiative w. acute renal failure - definition, outcome measures, animal models, fluid therapy and information technology needs: the second international consensus conference of the acute dialysis quality initiative (ADQI) group. Crit Care 2004; 8(4):R204–12.

4. Mehta RL, Kellum JA, Shah SV, et al. Acute Kidney Injury Network: report of an initiative to improve outcomes in acute kidney injury. Crit Care 2007; 11(2):R31.

5. KDIGO clinical practice guideline for the management of blood pressure in chronic kidney disease. Kidney Int 2012;2(5):85.

6. Katzberg RW, Haller C. Contrast-induced nephrotoxicity: clinical landscape. Kidney Int Suppl 2006;(100): S3–7. https://doi.org/10.1038/sj.ki.5000366.

7. Varc-3 Writing C, Genereux P, Piazza N, et al. Valve academic research consortium 3: updated endpoint definitions for aortic valve clinical research. J Am Coll Cardiol 2021;77(21):2717–46.

8. Mehran R, Nikolsky E. Contrast-induced nephropathy: definition, epidemiology, and patients at risk. Kidney Int Suppl 2006;(100):S11–5. https://doi.org/10.1038/sj.ki.5000368.

9. Amin AP, Bach RG, Caruso ML, et al. Association of variation in contrast volume with acute kidney injury in patients undergoing percutaneous coronary intervention. JAMA cardiology 2017;2(9):1007–12.

10. Wu MY, Lo WC, Wu YC, et al. The incidence of contrast-induced nephropathy and the need of dialysis in patients receiving angiography: a systematic review and meta-analysis. Front Med 2022;9:862534.

11. Schonenberger E, Martus P, Bosserdt M, et al. Kidney injury after intravenous versus intra-arterial contrast agent in patients suspected of having coronary artery disease: a randomized trial. Radiology 2019;292(3):664–72.

12. Lauver DA, Carey EG, Bergin IL, et al. Sildenafil citrate for prophylaxis of nephropathy in an animal model of contrast-induced acute kidney injury. PLoS One 2014;9(11):e113598.

13. Sendeski MM. Pathophysiology of renal tissue damage by iodinated contrast media. Clin Exp Pharmacol Physiol 2011;38(5):292–9.

14. Rackur H. New aspects of mechanism of action of povidone-iodine. J Hosp Infect 1985;6(Suppl A):13–23.

15. Hsu YC, Nomura S, Kruse CW. Some bactericidal and virucidal properties of iodine not affecting infectious RNA and DNA. Am J Epidemiol 1965; 82(3):317–28.

16. Dickenmann M, Oettl T, Mihatsch MJ. Osmotic nephrosis: acute kidney injury with accumulation of proximal tubular lysosomes due to administration of exogenous solutes. Am J Kidney Dis 2008;51(3):491–503.

17. Liss P, Persson PB, Hansell P, et al. Renal failure in 57 925 patients undergoing coronary procedures using iso-osmolar or low-osmolar contrast media. Kidney Int 2006;70(10):1811–7.

18. Haller C, Hizoh I. The cytotoxicity of iodinated radiocontrast agents on renal cells in vitro. Invest Radiol 2004;39(3):149–54.

19. Romano G, Briguori C, Quintavalle C, et al. Contrast agents and renal cell apoptosis. Eur Heart J 2008;29(20):2569–76.

20. Liu B, Chai Y, Guo W, et al. MicroRNA-188 aggravates contrast-induced apoptosis by targeting SRSF7 in novel isotonic contrast-induced acute kidney injury rat models and renal tubular epithelial cells. Ann Transl Med 2019;7(16):378.

21. Abrahams S, Greenwald L, Stetson DL. Contribution of renal medullary mitochondrial density to urinary concentrating ability in mammals. Am J Physiol 1991;261(3 Pt 2):R719–26.

22. Zou AP, Cowley AW Jr. Reactive oxygen species and molecular regulation of renal oxygenation. Acta Physiol Scand 2003;179(3):233–41.

23. Graier WF, Frieden M, Malli R. Mitochondria and Ca(2+) signaling: old guests, new functions. Pflueg Arch Eur J Physiol 2007;455(3):375–96.

24. Taylor CT. Mitochondria and cellular oxygen sensing in the HIF pathway. Biochem J 2008; 409(1):19–26.

25. Sun G, Kemble DJ. To C or not to C: direct and indirect redox regulation of Src protein tyrosine kinase. Cell Cycle 2009;8(15):2353–5.

26. Pisani A, Riccio E, Andreucci M, et al. Role of reactive oxygen species in pathogenesis of radiocontrast-induced nephropathy. BioMed Res Int 2013;2013:868321.

27. Persson PB, Hansell P, Liss P. Pathophysiology of contrast medium-induced nephropathy. Kidney Int 2005;68(1):14–22.

28. Heyman SN, Rosen S, Khamaisi M, et al. Reactive oxygen species and the pathogenesis of radiocontrast-induced nephropathy. Invest Radiol 2010;45(4):188–95.

29. Sendeski MM, Persson AB, Liu ZZ, et al. Iodinated contrast media cause endothelial damage leading to vasoconstriction of human and rat vasa recta. Am J Physiol Renal Physiol 2012;303(12):F1592–8.

30. Bakris GL, Lass N, Gaber AO, et al. Radiocontrast medium-induced declines in renal function: a role for oxygen free radicals. Am J Physiol 1990;258(1 Pt 2):F115–20.

31. Toprak O, Cirit M, Tanrisev M, et al. Preventive effect of nebivolol on contrast-induced nephropathy in rats. Nephrol Dial Transplant 2008;23(3):853–9.

32. Cetin M, Devrim E, Serin Kilicoglu S, et al. Ionic high-osmolar contrast medium causes oxidant

stress in kidney tissue: partial protective role of ascorbic acid. Ren Fail 2008;30(5):567–72.

33. Efrati S, Dishy V, Averbukh M, et al. The effect of N-acetylcysteine on renal function, nitric oxide, and oxidative stress after angiography. Kidney Int 2003;64(6):2182–7.

34. Baylis C. Sexual dimorphism in the aging kidney: differences in the nitric oxide system. Nat Rev Nephrol 2009;5(7):384–96.

35. Delp MD, Behnke BJ, Spier SA, et al. Ageing diminishes endothelium-dependent vasodilatation and tetrahydrobiopterin content in rat skeletal muscle arterioles. The Journal of physiology 2008;586(4): 1161–8.

36. Heyman SN, Rosenberger C, Rosen S, et al. Why is diabetes mellitus a risk factor for contrast-induced nephropathy? BioMed Res Int 2013;2013:123589.

37. Heyman SN, Reichman J, Brezis M. Pathophysiology of radiocontrast nephropathy: a role for medullary hypoxia. Invest Radiol 1999;34(11):685–91.

38. Pallone TL, Turner MR, Edwards A, et al. Countercurrent exchange in the renal medulla. Am J Physiol Regul Integr Comp Physiol 2003;284(5):R1153–75.

39. X-ray contrast media : overview, use and pharmaceutical aspects. Berlin, Heidelberg: Springer Berlin Heidelberg; 2018. Imprint: Springer.

40. Heyman SN, Rosenberger C, Rosen S. Regional alterations in renal haemodynamics and oxygenation: a role in contrast medium-induced nephropathy. Nephrol Dial Transplant 2005; 20(Suppl 1):i6–11.

41. Heyman SN, Rosen S, Rosenberger C. Renal parenchymal hypoxia, hypoxia adaptation, and the pathogenesis of radiocontrast nephropathy. Clin J Am Soc Nephrol 2008;3(1):288–96.

42. Sendeski M, Patzak A, Pallone TL, et al. Iodixanol, constriction of medullary descending vasa recta, and risk for contrast medium-induced nephropathy. Radiology 2009;251(3):697–704.

43. Armaly Z, Artol S, Jabbour AR, et al. Impact of pretreatment with carnitine and tadalafil on contrast-induced nephropathy in CKD patients. Ren Fail 2019;41(1):976–86.

44. Liu ZZ, Viegas VU, Perlewitz A, et al. Iodinated contrast media differentially affect afferent and efferent arteriolar tone and reactivity in mice: a possible explanation for reduced glomerular filtration rate. Radiology 2012;265(3):762–71.

45. Sendeski M, Patzak A, Persson PB. Constriction of the vasa recta, the vessels supplying the area at risk for acute kidney injury, by four different iodinated contrast media, evaluating ionic, nonionic, monomeric and dimeric agents. Invest Radiol 2010;45(8):453–7.

46. Eng J, Wilson RF, Subramaniam RM, et al. Comparative effect of contrast media type on the incidence of contrast-induced nephropathy: a systematic review and meta-analysis. Annals of internal medicine 2016;164(6):417–24.

47. Hoang K, Tan JC, Derby G, et al. Determinants of glomerular hypofiltration in aging humans. Kidney Int 2003;64(4):1417–24.

48. Weinstein JR, Anderson S. The aging kidney: physiological changes. Adv Chron Kidney Dis 2010; 17(4):302–7.

49. Schrier RW. Role of diminished renal function in cardiovascular mortality: marker or pathogenetic factor? J Am Coll Cardiol 2006;47(1):1–8.

50. Tsai TT, Patel UD, Chang TI, et al. Contemporary incidence, predictors, and outcomes of acute kidney injury in patients undergoing percutaneous coronary interventions: insights from the NCDR Cath-PCI registry. JACC Cardiovasc Interv 2014; 7(1):1–9.

51. Mohebi R, Karimi Galougahi K, Garcia JJ, et al. Long-term clinical impact of contrast-associated acute kidney injury following PCI: an ADAPT-DES substudy. JACC Cardiovasc Interv 2022;15(7): 753–66.

52. Gruberg L, Mintz GS, Mehran R, et al. The prognostic implications of further renal function deterioration within 48 h of interventional coronary procedures in patients with pre-existent chronic renal insufficiency. J Am Coll Cardiol 2000;36(5):1542–8.

53. McCullough PA, Adam A, Becker CR, et al. Epidemiology and prognostic implications of contrast-induced nephropathy. Am J Cardiol 2006;98(6A): 5K–13K.

54. Dangas G, Iakovou I, Nikolsky E, et al. Contrast-induced nephropathy after percutaneous coronary interventions in relation to chronic kidney disease and hemodynamic variables. Am J Cardiol 2005; 95(1):13–9.

55. Nemoto N, Iwasaki M, Nakanishi M, et al. Impact of continuous deterioration of kidney function 6 to 8 months after percutaneous coronary intervention for acute coronary syndrome. Am J Cardiol 2014; 113(10):1647–51.

56. Aubry P, Brillet G, Catella L, et al. Outcomes, risk factors and health burden of contrast-induced acute kidney injury: an observational study of one million hospitalizations with image-guided cardiovascular procedures. BMC Nephrol 2016;17(1):167.

57. Subramanian S, Tumlin J, Bapat B, et al. Economic burden of contrast-induced nephropathy: implications for prevention strategies. J Med Econ 2007; 10(2):119–34.

58. McDonald RJ, McDonald JS, Carter RE, et al. Intravenous contrast material exposure is not an independent risk factor for dialysis or mortality. Radiology 2014;273(3):714–25.

59. Bruce RJ, Djamali A, Shinki K, et al. Background fluctuation of kidney function versus contrast-

induced nephrotoxicity. AJR Am J Roentgenol 2009;192(3):711–8.

60. Davenport MS, Khalatbari S, Cohan RH, et al. Contrast material-induced nephrotoxicity and intravenous low-osmolality iodinated contrast material: risk stratification by using estimated glomerular filtration rate. Radiology 2013;268(3):719–28.

61. Wilhelm-Leen E, Montez-Rath ME, Chertow G. Estimating the risk of radiocontrast-associated nephropathy. J Am Soc Nephrol 2017;28(2):653–9.

62. Newhouse JH, Kho D, Rao QA, et al. Frequency of serum creatinine changes in the absence of iodinated contrast material: implications for studies of contrast nephrotoxicity. AJR Am J Roentgenol 2008;191(2):376–82.

Predicting Contrast-induced Renal Complications

Emily A. Eitzman[a], Rachel G. Kroll, BS[a],
Prasanthi Yelavarthy, MD[b],
Nadia R. Sutton, MD, MPH[c,d,*]

KEYWORDS

- Chronic kidney disease • Percutaneous coronary intervention • Contrast-induced nephropathy
- Contrast media • Risk-prediction

KEY POINTS

- Identification of patients vulnerable to the development of renal complications is an initial critical step in preventing renal impairment and a new need for dialysis after contrast exposure.
- Contrast media volume, age and sex of the patient, a history of chronic kidney disease and/or diabetes, clinical presentation, and hemodynamic and hydration status are factors known to predict incident contrast-associated nephropathy.
- Many risk models have been created using pre- and post-procedural factors to predict the future risk of contrast-induced nephropathy and a new need for dialysis.
- Online calculators such as the SCAI Risk Assessment Tool can be utilized to categorize the patient risk of contrast-associated kidney injury and a new requirement for dialysis.

INTRODUCTION

Chronic kidney disease (CKD) is an independent risk factor for the development of coronary artery disease (CAD) and overlaps with other risk factors such as hypertension and diabetes which lead to both CKD and CAD.[1] The presence of CAD in patient populations can be asymptomatic, or can manifest symptoms ranging from stable angina to acute coronary syndromes (myocardial infarction), cardiogenic shock, and cardiac arrest.[2] Currently, determining the presence of obstructive CAD requires the use of contrast media (CM), either using non-invasive (computer tomography) or minimally-invasive (coronary angiogram) approaches. In addition to medical therapy, percutaneous coronary intervention (PCI) is a minimally invasive approach to restoring myocardial blood flow using angioplasty and /or coronary artery stenting.[3] Depending on the clinical circumstances, this procedure is used to reduce symptoms due to coronary artery stenoses and/or reduce the risk of future death and myocardial infarction.[4]

PCI, except under rare circumstances, utilizes intra-arterial CM in order to opacify coronary arteries in the cardiac catheterization laboratory.[5] CM has the potential to negatively impact renal function, and patients with pre-existing chronic kidney disease are more susceptible to this effect.[6] Once it has been determined that an individual could benefit from a heart catheterization requiring CM, identifying those at risk for contrast-associated kidney injury (CA-AKI, now

---

[a] Cardiovascular Research Center, 7301A MSRB III, 1150 West Medical Center Drive, Ann Arbor, MI 48109-0644, USA; [b] Munson Medical Center, Traverse City, MI, USA; [c] Department of Internal Medicine, Division of Cardiovascular Medicine, Vanderbilt University Medical Center, Nashville, TN, USA; [d] Department of Biomedical Engineering, Vanderbilt University, Nashville, TN, USA
* Corresponding author. Vanderbilt University Medical Center, Preston Research Building 360, 2220 Pierce Avenue, Nashville, TN 37232.
E-mail address: nadia.sutton@vumc.org

Intervent Cardiol Clin 12 (2023) 499–513
https://doi.org/10.1016/j.iccl.2023.06.001
2211-7458/23/© 2023 Elsevier Inc. All rights reserved.

a favored term over earlier contrast-induced nephropathy [CIN] is a key initial step in preventing this complication. Systemic clinical application of prediction models for the development of renal complications of PCI raise awareness of an individual patient's risk of CA-AKI. Patients at increased risk can receive targeted interventions to reduce the risk of renal complications after PCI which can potentially be used to monitor the quality and safety of PCI. Since renal complications of PCI are associated with other poor outcome measures, predicting and preventing renal complications of CM exposure are critical to performing PCI safely. In this article, we will describe available risk prediction equations after initial discussion about risk factors associated with CA-AKI (Fig. 1).

RISK FACTORS FOR CONTRAST-ASSOCIATED ACUTE KIDNEY INJURY

Patient age and sex

Age is a leading risk factor for the development of renal complications after contrast exposure.[7–12] The risk of AKI due to contrast rises with age, beginning in patients 50 years of age and increasing steadily through age greater than 90.[10] Patients ≥ 73 years of age are three times more likely than younger patients to develop CA-AKI,[13] while patients ≥ 80 years have an odds ratio of 19.6 for the development of serious renal dysfunction after contrast exposure, relative to patients less than 50 years of age.[14] The AGEF (age and ejection fraction ratio) score for the prediction of CA-AKI in patients being treated for ST-elevation myocardial infarction (STEMI) includes only three clinical variables: age, ejection fraction, and estimated glomerular filtration rate (eGFR).[11]

Females have odds of developing renal complications after contrast exposure that is 1.5 to 2.0 times that of males.[14,15] Further, females without a history of CKD that develop CA-AKI have a higher risk of 1-year mortality.[16] The mechanism underlying the independent association between patient sex or age and renal dysfunction after contrast exposure is unclear and requires further study.

Chronic kidney disease

Patients with CKD undergoing PCI carry a higher risk of serious complications of PCI, including mortality.[17,18] Tajti and colleagues described significantly higher rates of in-hospital mortality and major adverse cardiovascular events after PCI in patients with CKD versus those without CKD. Patients with renal dysfunction have a higher risk of requiring repeat urgent revascularization.[19] CKD increases the risk of multiple PCI complications, including the development of CA-AKI.

Pre-existing CKD is the most significant risk factor in the development of CA-AKI (Fig. 1).[20] Beginning with a baseline eGFR less than 60 mL/min per 1.73 m^2, progressively lower eGFR rates are associated with an increasingly greater risk of CA-AKI.[6,18] For example, with an eGFR of 30 mL/min per 1.73 m^2, the risk of developing CA-AKI is as high as 30% to 40%, compared to a risk of 2% for the general population.[18,21]

Diabetes mellitus

Diabetes often exists concurrently with conditions such as acute coronary syndromes, that lead to PCI; approximately 1 in 3 patients undergoing PCI have diabetes.[15,22,23] Diabetic patients have a higher risk of developing AKI after PCI compared to their non-diabetic counterparts.[15,24,25] The physiologic mechanisms behind this correlation include increased renal oxygen consumption and reduced medullary oxygenation induced by diabetes combined with reduced renal perfusion triggered by CM.[26] Together, this leads to renal hypoxia, impairing kidney function. Hyperglycemia due to diabetes may also be an independent predictor of CA-AKI. The incidence of CA-AKI was reported as being significantly higher among diabetic patients with serum glucose ≥ 150 mg/dL compared to non-hyperglycemic patients.[27]

Clinical presentation

Myocardial infarction is associated with post-PCI CA-AKI.[28] In several studies, presentation with STEMI was shown to independently predict AKI post-PCI.[10,22] In their analysis of 985,737 patients who underwent PCI, Tsai and colleagues observed a higher incidence of AKI post-PCI in patients who presented with non-STEMI or STEMI when compared with other indications for PCI.[22] Similarly, in their retrospective analysis using the Mayo Clinic PCI registry, Rihal and colleagues reported that acute myocardial infarction within 24 hours before the index PCI, unstable angina, and prior myocardial infarction were all associated with CA-AKI post-PCI.[24] More than half of patients who ultimately experienced CA-AKI initially presented with unstable angina.[24] The incidence of CA-AKI in patients with STEMI undergoing primary PCI with a Killip Class II presentation is greater than the risk of CA-AKI in patients undergoing elective PCI.[29] Impaired left ventricular function (ejection fraction < 40%) at the time of PCI is also associated with development of CA-AKI.[11,28,30,31]

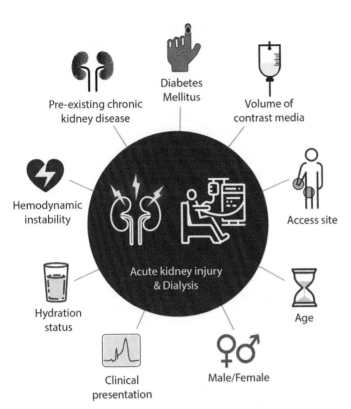

Fig. 1. Risk factors for the development of acute kidney injury and new requirement for dialysis following contrast medium exposure.[20]

Hemodynamic instability

Periprocedural hemodynamic instability, indicated by hypotension, requirement for vasopressors, or use of mechanical support devices, is associated with an increased risk of CA-AKI in patients undergoing PCI.[15,28,30–32] This association between hemodynamic instability and increased risk of CA-AKI is likely multifactorial, related to vasoconstriction and cardiogenic shock resulting in low cardiac output, and the downstream impact on renal perfusion (see Lalith Vemireddy and Shweta Bansal's article, "Contrast-Associated Acute Kidney Injury: Definitions, Epidemiology, Pathophysiology and Implications," in this issue).

Volume status

CM concentration in the renal medulla correlates with cytotoxicity, and volume expansion with saline has been shown to reduce the risk of subsequent CA-AKI.[33] However, pre-procedure hydration status based on a physical examination can be challenging to predict. In addition, emergent procedures utilizing CM in the setting of hypovolemia or loss of blood volume are sometimes required. Anemia is known to be associated with acute kidney injury after PCI in patients with and without pre-existing kidney disease.[34] Further, peri-procedural bleeding results in anemia, volume depletion, and potentially hemodynamic instability compounding CA-AKI.[35] In these cases, expeditious volume resuscitation and minimization of contrast exposure are important preventive interventions.

Access site

Recent studies have suggested that a radial arterial access site for coronary intervention and angiography carry a lower risk of bleeding and major vascular complications when compared with femoral arterial access.[36–38] In addition, observational and randomized studies have demonstrated that AKI occurs less frequently in patients who undergo invasive procedures with CM via the radial artery access when compared to patients who have their procedure performed via the femoral artery.[39,40] Proposed explanations include that radial access is accompanied by a lower risk of renal atherosclerotic embolization and peri-procedural bleeding avoiding hypovolemia. Radial access has been historically avoided in patients with CKD who may need future hemodialysis, although practice patterns may be shifting.[38]

Volume of contrast media

The volume of CM administered to patients in a single setting or during multiple administrations within a short duration is strongly associated with the incidence of CA-AKI (see Fig. 1).[20] CM becomes more concentrated in the hyperosmolar environment of the renal tubules. This increased fluid viscosity reduces renal blood flow, subsequently inducing hypoxia of the renal medulla and cell death due to higher contact time between the cytotoxic CM and endothelial cells.[41]

Risk models have been proposed to predict renal complications of PCI (Table 1) that can be applied in clinical settings, utilizing CM volume and either calculated creatinine clearance (CCC) or eGFR. The incidence of CA-AKI has been found to increase when the CM volume/eGFR ratio surpasses 1.[42–44] Similarly, a CM volume (mL) to CCC (mL/min) ratio exceeding 2 is associated with an increased risk of CA-AKI with ratios greater than 3 linked with substantially increased risk.[45–48]

Predictive formulas for the maximum safe CM dose have been proposed.[49–51] Contrast volume for ultra-low contrast angiography is defined as a contrast volume/eGFR ratio of $\leq$ 1.[52,53] Zero-contrast PCI has been performed as well, harnessing the ability to perform intravascular ultrasound imaging without contrast.[5,54,55] Additional strategies such as using saline rather than contrast for optical coherence tomography-guided PCI have also been described.[56] CO_2 angiography is not accompanied by renal toxicity but is contraindicated for PCI due to the risk of gas embolism, neurotoxicity, and cerebral infarction.[57]

Special populations

The patient population undergoing evaluation for renal transplant that is not yet on dialysis presents unique challenges to health professionals who are faced with determining whether the benefits of PCI outweigh the risks. It is not uncommon in this population for a patient with a GFR less than 15 mL/min per 1.73 m^2 to require PCI due to perceived excessive surgical risk for renal transplantation without intervention. A recent study of 535 renal transplant recipients found that pre-transplant PCI was associated with a reduced incidence of adverse post-transplant coronary events, but the association did not reach statistical significance ($P = .06$).[58] In another study, renal transplant candidates with CKD for whom coronary intervention was recommended but not performed, experienced a higher mortality rate.[59] Other studies have found no difference in mortality between renal transplant candidates who undergo coronary angiography or PCI and those who do not, suggesting that it may be safer for renal transplant candidates to abstain from these procedures.[60,61] Further studies will be helpful to

understanding whether the risk of worsening renal function with PCI and potentially expediting a requirement for dialysis is outweighed by the benefit of undergoing renal transplantation with a reduced risk of cardiovascular complications.

RENAL COMPLICATIONS OF CONTRAST EXPOSURE

Acute kidney injury

The definition of AKI due to any cause has been defined variably in the literature, ranging from a change in serum creatinine level or change in urine output, to a need for dialysis.[62] Several staging systems have been proposed to provide a consensus definition of AKI, among them the Acute Kidney Injury Network (AKIN) and the Acute Dialysis Quality Initiative (ADQI) systems, both of which use change in serum creatinine or urine output to stratify varied levels of renal failure.[62,63] (see Gudsoorkar and Colleague's article, "Definition, Staging, and Role of Biomarkers in Acute Kidney Injury in the Context of Cardiovascular Interventions," in this issue). outlines all the definition in detail. When considering CA-AKI specifically, prediction models have utilized varying definitions of post-PCI AKI, including an increase in serum creatinine of either $\geq$ 25% or $\geq$ 50%, $\geq$ 0.5 mg/dL, and $\geq$ 1.0 mg/dL. Despite these varying definitions, prediction models may be comparable even when CA-AKI definitions differ slightly. Capodanno and colleagues reported that a CM volume to estimated creatinine clearance ratio $\geq$ 4 reliably predicted the risk of CA-AKI regardless of the definition (either increase in serum creatinine $\geq$ 0.5 mg/dL or $\geq$ 25%).[64] In the absence of a universal definition of AKI, prediction models can be evaluated through comparison of c-statistics; validated models with a c-statistic of 0.8 or greater could be acceptable for use in practice, if the variables are readily accessible.[65]

New-onset dialysis

Development of a need for dialysis due to CA-AKI is correlated with extended duration of hospitalization, long-term renal impairment, and increased short- and long-term mortality rates.[14,18,66] Ultimately, reducing the risk of CA-AKI also reduces this more serious complication of newly requiring dialysis, and five different risk models have been designed to predict, specifically, the need for dialysis.[10,12,14,18,66] All of these models include pre-existing impaired renal function and diabetes as risk factors for requiring dialysis post-PCI. Several models also noted an association between hemodynamic instability and a new need for dialysis post-PCI.[10,12,14,66]

Table 1
Prediction scores for renal complications after PCI using pre-procedural characteristics

First Author	Population	Outcomes Predicted	Model Variables	Cut-Offs	Test Characteristics
Duan et al,[8] 2017	Derivation set 1076 Validation set 701	CA-AKI (≥50% or ≥ 0.3 mg/dL serum creatinine increase from baseline within 48 h)	Age >75 y, serum creatinine levels, NT-proBNP, hs-CRP, primary PCI	Low risk (0–8) Moderate risk (9–17) High risk (18–26) Very-high risk (≥27)	Prospective observational, single center
Chen et al,[9] 2014	Derivation set 1500 Validation set 1000	CA-AKI (≥25% or ≥ 0.5 mg/dL serum creatinine increase)	Age ≥70, history of MI, diabetes, hypotension, LVEF ≤ 45%, anemia, eGFR < 60, HDL <1mmol/L, urgent PCI	Low risk (<7) Moderate risk (8–12) High risk (13–16) Very high risk (≥17)	Retrospective, observational, single center in China
Tsai et al,[10] 2014	Derivation set 662,504 Validation set 284,508	CA-AKI (≥50% or ≥ 0.3mg/dL 50% serum creatinine increase) and new-onset dialysis	Age, prior 2 wk HF, GFR, diabetes, prior HF/CVD, NSTEMI/UA, STEMI, prior card shock or cardiac arrest, anemia, IABP		Retrospective, observational, multicenter (1253 sites using NCDR Cath/PCI registry)
Ando et al,[11] 2013	481 consecutive patients with STEMI	CA-AKI (≥25% or ≥ 0.5mg/dL serum creatinine increase)	AGEF score (Adding 1 point to the Age/EF(%) ratio if the eGFR was <60mL/min)		Prospective, observational, single-center study
Gurm et al,[12] 2013	Derivation set 40,001 Validation set 20,572	CA-AKI (≥0.5 mg/dL serum creatinine increase) and new onset dialysis	PCI indication/status, CAD presentation, cardiogenic shock, heart failure, pre-PCI LVEF, diabetes, age, weight, height, CK-MD, creatinine, hemoglobin, Troponin I, and troponin T		Retrospective, observational, multicenter (all non-federal hospitals in Michigan using BMC2 registry)
Maioli et al,[13] 2010	1218 consecutive patients undergoing PCI (excluding STEMI)	CA-AKI (≥0.5mg/dL)	Age > 73, diabetes, LVEF ≤ 45%, creatinine ≥ 1.5mg/dL or CrCl ≤ 44mL/min, post-hydration Cr	Low risk (≤3) Moderate risk (4–6) High risk (7–8) Very high risk (≥9)	Prospective, observational, single study in Italy

(continued on next page)

Table 1
(continued)

First Author	Population	Outcomes Predicted	Cut-Offs	Model Variables	Test Characteristics
Brown et al,[14] 2008	11,141 consecutive patients undergoing PCI	CA-AKI (≥50% or ≥ 2.0 mg/dL serum creatinine increase) or new dialysis	Risk score 0-37.5	Age ≥ 80, female, diabetes, urgent/emergent, CHF, creatinine, pre-PCI IABP	Prospective, observational using the Northern New England Cardiovascular Disease Study Group (NNECDSG)
Freeman et al,[66] 2002	Derivation set 10,729 Validation set 5863	New-onset dialysis		Peripheral artery disease, diabetes, CKD (Cr > 2mg/dL), heart failure, cardiogenic shock	Prospective multicenter using BMC2 registry (8 academic and community hospitals in Michigan)
McCullough et al,[18] 1997	Derivation set 1869 Validation set 1826	New-onset dialysis		CrCl, diabetes, expected contrast dose	Prospective observational, single center
Mehran et al,[70] 2021	Derivation set 14,616 Validation set 5606	CA-AKI		Clinical presentation, estimated glomerular filtration rate, left ventricular ejection fraction, diabetes, hemoglobin, basal glucose, congestive heart failure, age	Prospective observational, single center
Li et al,[79] 2022	4295 patients undergoing coronary angiography	CA-AKI	MRCD = 5mL x bodyweight (kg)/serum creatinine (mg/dL)	Age, gender, hemoglobin, N-terminal of the prohormone brain natriuretic peptide, neutrophil-to-lymphocyte ratio, cardiac troponin I, loop diuretics use	Prospective observational, single center

Abbreviations: BMC2, blue cross blue shield of michigan cardiovascular consortium; BNP, B-type natriuretic peptide; CA-AKI, Contrast-associated acute kidney injury; CHF, congestive heart failure; CK-MB, creatine kinase-MB; cr, creatine; CrCl, creatinine clearance; CRP, C-reactive protein; CVD, cardiovascular disease; HDL, high-density lipoprotein; HF, heart failure; hs, high-sensitivity; IABP, intra-aortic balloon pump; LVEF, left ventricular ejection fraction; MRCD, maximum radiographic contrast dose; NCDR, national cardiovascular data repository; NSTEMI, non-ST-elevation myocardial infarction; NT, N-terminal; UA, unstable angina.

PREDICTION TOOLS FOR RISK CALCULATION

Many prediction models have been developed to predict post-PCI renal complications. These risk scores can be divided into 2 groups: those risk scores including pre-procedural characteristics (see Table 1) and those including both pre- and post-procedural characteristics (Table 2). The risk scores with the pre-procedural characteristics can be used as a tool to assess the risk of renal complications before the PCI is performed and be used to help guide practice decisions for patients undergoing PCI minimizing the risk of development of AKI, especially for those with CKD. The risk scores including post-procedural characteristics take into account contrast dose, useful in guiding strategies for contrast volume reduction and potentially for assessing quality. There is considerable overlap in the risk factors that were used to develop these scores.

Comparison of risk scores

In risk models, prediction rules with a c-statistic greater than 0.80 are generally considered acceptable for application in daily practice.[65] The predictive value of the scores in CA-AKI prediction studies vary, with c-statistics between 0.68 and 0.89. External validation by another research group is an important next step undertaken prior to application to clinical practice to ensure that the findings of a study can be generalized to other contexts. Three risk scores have undergone rigorous validation in external cohorts. For example, the risk score by Mehran and colleagues from 2004 has been validated in 4 studies, with c-statistics ranging between 0.57 and 0.85.[67–69] A more recent model called the Mehran-2 CA-AKI Risk Score resulted in a higher c-statistic of 0.86.[70] The score by Bartholomew and colleagues has been validated in 2 additional studies; however, the predictive score varied between these 2 validation studies.[71] Use of different definitions of post-PCI AKI from the original study was likely the cause of conflicting results limiting the interpretability.

Prediction of acute kidney injury and new-onset dialysis post-percutaneous coronary intervention

Eighteen of the 20 studies were developed to predict AKI (see Tables 1 and 2). However, the definition of AKI post-PCI varies between studies (increase in serum creatinine >25%, > 50%, >0.3 mg/dL, > 0.5 mg/dL, >1.0 mg/dL, > 2.0 mg/dL or a combination of 2 of the above) making direct comparisons challenging. There are 5 risk tools

that have been developed for the prediction of new-onset dialysis post-PCI. Of these, the risk score by McCullough et al contains contrast dose and therefore cannot be used pre-procedurally.[18] The risk scores by Freeman and colleagues[66] and Gurm and colleagues[12] utilize baseline patient characteristics, lending the models well to pre-procedural prediction of new-onset dialysis post-PCI. Employing these risk prediction tools to target preventative strategies to high-risk patients systematically provides an opportunity for improved safety and reduced risk of diagnostic angiograms and PCI. Thus far, utilization of these tools has been associated with reduction in contrast volume; however, the impact on incidence of CA-AKI or other clinical outcomes has yet to be documented.

High performing models

Of the numerous models that are available to predict the risk of CA-AKI, the scores by Tsai and colleagues, Gurm and colleagues, and Mehran and colleagues have the largest derivation and validation sets.[10,12,70] The models use pre-procedural characteristics, making it useful to help patients make informed decisions about undergoing a PCI. Several organizations have developed online risk calculators using these models simplifying the process for clinicians to calculate risk (Table 3). Of these 4 calculators using pre-procedures variables, Society for Cardiovascular Angiography and Interventions Foundation (SCAI) PCI risk calculator has been the latest, rigorously tested, and most widely used. This model extends the work described by Gurm and colleagues[12] and computes the risk of in-hospital mortality, femoral vascular injury, bleeding, transfusion, 1-year target vessel revascularization, and 30-day readmission in addition to dialysis and CA-AKI. Among the risk calculators using additional post-procedural variables, the score by Mehran and colleagues[15] is the most widely used; this score is also simple and practical in the clinical setting (see Table 3).

A more recent study by Mehran and colleagues[70] (Mehran-2 CA-AKI risk score) has provided additional insight regarding predictors for CA-AKI. In this study, the derivation cohort comprised patients who underwent PCI between 2012 and 2017 and the validation cohort comprised of patients who underwent PCI between 2018 and 2020.[70] It was found that for both the derivation and validation cohort, inclusion of both pre-procedural and procedural variables enhanced the c-statistic for predicting CA-AKI significantly compared to inclusion of only pre-procedural variables.[70] The pre-procedural

Table 2
Prediction scores for renal complications after PCI using post-procedural characteristics

	2867 Consecutive patients Undergoing PCI	CA-AKI (≥25% or ≥0.5mg/dL Serum Creatinine Increase)	Contrast Volume/creatinine Clearance	V/CrCl Ratio ≥ 6.15 Associated with Increased risk of CIN	Prospective, Observational, Single Center in Italy
Barbieri 2016[80]					
Victor et al,[81] 2014	Derivation set 900 Validation set 300	CA-AKI (≥50% or ≥ 0.5 mg/dL serum creatinine increase)	GFR, contrast volume, hemoglobin, diabetic microangiopathy, hypotension, albuminuria, peripheral vascular disease		Prospective, observational, single center in India
Tziakas et al,[82] 2013	Derivation set 488 Validation set 200	CA-AKI (≥25% or ≥ 0.5mg/dL serum creatinine increase)	CKD, metformin use, prior PCI, peripheral arterial disease, contrast volume ≥ 300mL	Low risk (≤2 points) High risk (>2 points)	Prospective, observational, single center in Greece
Chong et al,[83] 2012	770 consecutive patients undergoing PCI	CA-AKI (≥25% or ≥ 0.5mg/dL serum creatinine increase)	Age, eGFR, post-PCI CK (for every 500 U/L increase), contrast volume	Low risk (1–3) Moderate risk (4–6) High risk (7–8) Extremely high risk (≥9)	Prospective, observational, single center in Singapore
Tan et al,[84] 2012	1140 consecutive patients undergoing PCI	CA-AKI (≥0.5mg/dL serum creatinine increase)	Contrast volume/creatinine clearance	V/CrCl ratio > 2.62 associated with increased risk of CIN	Prospective, observational, single center in China
Fu et al,[85] 2012	Derivation set 668 Validation set 277	CA-AKI (≥25% or ≥ 0.5mg/dL serum creatinine increase)	eGFR, diabetes, LVEF <45%, hypotension, age > 70, MI, emergency PCI, anemia, contrast volume > 200mL	Low risk (≤4) Moderate risk (5–8) High risk (9–12) Very high risk (≥13)	Retrospective, observational, single center in China
Ghani et al,[86] 2009	Derivation set 247 Validation set 100	CA-AKI (≥25% or ≥ 0.5 mg/dL serum creatinine increase)	Creatinine, shock, female gender, multiple vessel stenting, diabetes	Low (≤4) Moderate (5–8) High (9–12) Very high (≥12)	Prospective, observational, single center in Kuwait

Study	Population / Sample	Outcome	Predictors	Risk categories	Study design
Mehran et al,[15] 2004	Derivation set 5571 Validation set 2786	CA-AKI (≥25% or ≥0.5 mg/dL serum creatinine increase)	Hypotension, heart failure, CKD, diabetes, age > 75 y, anemia, IABP, contrast volume	Low risk ≤ 5 Moderate risk 6–10 High risk 11–15 Very high risk ≥ 16	Prospective observational, using Cardiovascular Research Foundation (CRF database)
Marenzi et al,[28] 2004	208 consecutive AMI patients	CA-AKI (≥0.5 mg/dL serum creatinine increase)	Age > 75 y, anterior infarction, time-to-reperfusion, contrast volume, use of IABP	Risk score 1–5	Prospective observational, single center
Bartholomew et al,[32] 2004	Derivation set 10,481 Validation set 9998	CA-AKI (≥1.0 mg/dL serum creatinine increase)	eGFR < 60mL/min, IABP, urgent/emergent procedure, diabetes, heart failure, hypertension, peripheral artery disease, contrast volume > 260mL	Low risk 0–4 Moderate risk 5–6 High risk 7–8 Very high risk 9–11	Prospective observational, single center
Mehran et al,[70] 2021	Derivation set 14,616 Validation set 5606	CA-AKI	Clinical presentation, estimated glomerular filtration rate, left ventricular ejection fraction, diabetes, hemoglobin, basal glucose, congestive heart failure, age, contrast volume, peri-procedural bleeding, no flow or slow flow post-procedure, complex PCI anatomy		Observational, single center

Abbreviations: CA-AKI, Contrast-associated acute kidney injury; CK, creatine kinase; CKD, chronic kidney disease; CrCl, creatinine clearance; GFR, glomerular filtration rate; IABP, intra-aortic balloon pump; PCI, percutaneous coronary interventions; V, volume.

Table 3
Online calculators to assess risks of peri-procedural complications

Name	Outcomes	Website	Pre or Post-procedural	c-statistic for AKI	c-statistic for Dialysis
BMC2 PCI risk calculator based on work by Gurm et al[12]	Estimated risk of death, blood transfusion, CA-AKI, and need for new dialysis	https://bmc2.org/calculators/multi	Pre-procedural	0.84	0.88
SCAI Risk Assessment Tool – extended the work by Gurm et al[12] Another SCAI tool uses the NCDR, MassDAC, and DELTA model	Risk of in-hospital mortality, transfusion, and CA-AKI In-hospital mortality, femoral vascular injury, bleeding, dialysis, CA-AKI, (AKI and dialysis given as an odds ratio vs a healthy 50-year-old), 1-year target vessel revascularization, and 30-d readmission.	http://scaipciriskapp.org/porc	Pre-procedural (for AKI and need for new dialysis)		
Protected PCI Community AKI calculator using Mehran score[15]	Risk of CA-AKI and risk of dialysis	https://www.heartrecovery.com/resources/calculators/acute-kidney-injury	Pre- and post-procedural	0.67	
NCDR AKI and Dialysis Risk after PCI based on work by Tsai et al,[10]	Risk of AKI and risk of dialysis	https://qxmd.com/calculate/calculator_386	Pre-procedural	0.71	0.88

Abbreviations: CA-AKI, Contrast-associated acute kidney injury; MassDAC, massachusetts data analysis center; NCDR, national cardiovascular data registry; PCI, percutaneous coronary interventions; SCAI, society for cardiovascular angiography and interventions.

variables included in this study were clinical presentation, eGFR, left ventricular ejection fraction, diabetes, hemoglobin, basal glucose, congestive heart failure, and age. The procedural variables were contrast volume, peri-procedural bleeding, no flow or slow flow post-procedure, and complex PCI anatomy.[70] The validation cohort resulted in the highest c-statistics with a c-statistic of 0.84 when only pre-procedural variables were analyzed and a c-statistic of 0.86 when procedural variables were also considered, confirming the relevance of including procedural variables when predicting CA-AKI.[70]

NOVEL APPROACHES
Biomarkers for the prediction of contrast-induced nephropathy

Biomarkers aside from eGFR and creatinine may be of interest in predicting CA-AKI. A recent study found that increased levels of high-sensitivity C-reactive protein and procalcitonin drawn prior to PCI are associated with a risk of CA-AKI post-PCI.[72] C-reactive protein and procalcitonin are proteins synthesized under stress conditions, and they play roles in inflammatory responses. Neutrophil gelatinase-associated lipocalin (NGAL), a glycoprotein stored in neutrophils and released when nephrons are inflamed or injured, is also associated with renal injury and a need for hemodialysis when drawn prior to PCI.[73] This study found that while serum levels of creatinine and blood urea nitrogen (BUN) could not detect early development of CA-AKI, serum levels of NGAL at 6 hours post-PCI could predict a future need for dialysis. Urinary adiponectin (UAPN) measured before angiography was also associated with CA-AKI with the area under the curve of adiponectin being greater than that of creatinine, indicating that urinary adiponectin may be more likely to predict CA-AKI than a patient's baseline creatinine level.[74] Another biomarker that has been found to have potential to predict CA-AKI is heat shock protein 27, which plays a role in protecting the kidney from cellular stress.[75] A recent study evaluated the biomarkers kidney injury molecule-1, interleukin-18, osteopontin, and cystatin C and determined that biomarker-enhanced risk models greatly enhance the prediction of CA-AKI.[76]

Electronic medical records and artificial intelligence to predict contrast-induced nephropathy

Electronic health records-based contrast limit tools have been evaluated and found to be associated with a decrease in contrast use during PCI and predict CA-AKI.[77]

Neural network-based models have also been discovered to be of use for predicting complications post-PCI such as AKI, bleeding, and death, though further research is needed to utilize these models in clinical practice.[78]

SUMMARY

Prediction of renal complications of contrast exposure is critical to targeting risk-reduction strategies including pre- and post-procedural hydration, strict contrast volume exposure limits, staging of procedures, and access site choice. Identifying patients vulnerable to this complication using readily available risk-prediction tools is an initial step toward reducing the risk of CA-AKI and a new need for dialysis. A clear understanding of risk factors for CA-AKI also helps identify effective preventive strategies. We recommend the SCAI Risk Assessment Tool to predict patient subgroups at the highest risk for CA-AKI to guide the treatment strategies.

CLINICS CARE POINTS

- Risk models have been developed to identify patients at high risk of developing contrast-associated kidney injury.
- Identification of patients at risk aids in the implementation of interventions to reduce the risk of developing contrast-associated acute kidney injury.

REFERENCES

1. Sarnak MJ, Amann K, Bangalore S, et al. Chronic Kidney Disease and Coronary Artery Disease: JACC State-of-the-Art Review. J Am Coll Cardiol 2019;74(14):1823–38.
2. Libby P, Theroux P. Pathophysiology of coronary artery disease. Circulation 2005;111(25):3481–8.
3. Sutton NR, Seth M, Madder RD, et al. Comparative Safety of Bioabsorbable Polymer Everolimus-Eluting, Durable Polymer Everolimus-Eluting, and Durable Polymer Zotarolimus-Eluting Stents in Contemporary Clinical Practice. Circ Cardiovasc Interv 2021;14(3):e009850.
4. Lawton JS, Tamis-Holland JE, Bangalore S, et al. 2021 ACC/AHA/SCAI Guideline for Coronary Artery Revascularization: Executive Summary: A Report of the American College of Cardiology/American Heart Association Joint Committee on Clinical Practice Guidelines. Circulation 2022;145(3):e4–17.

5. Ali ZA, Karimi Galougahi K, Nazif T, et al. Imaging- and physiology-guided percutaneous coronary intervention without contrast administration in advanced renal failure: a feasibility, safety, and outcome study. Eur Heart J 2016;37(40):3090–5.

6. Mehran R, Nikolsky E. Contrast-induced nephropathy: definition, epidemiology, and patients at risk. Kidney Int Suppl 2006;(100):S11–5.

7. Maioli M, Toso A, Leoncini M, et al. Persistent renal damage after contrast-induced acute kidney injury: incidence, evolution, risk factors, and prognosis. Circulation 2012;125(25):3099–107.

8. Duan C, Cao Y, Liu Y, et al. A New Preprocedure Risk Score for Predicting Contrast-Induced Acute Kidney Injury. Can J Cardiol 2017;33(6):714–23.

9. Chen YL, Fu NK, Xu J, et al. A simple preprocedural score for risk of contrast-induced acute kidney injury after percutaneous coronary intervention. Catheter Cardiovasc Interv 2014;83(1):E8–16.

10. Tsai TT, Patel UD, Chang TI, et al. Validated contemporary risk model of acute kidney injury in patients undergoing percutaneous coronary interventions: insights from the National Cardiovascular Data Registry Cath-PCI Registry. J Am Heart Assoc 2014;3(6):e001380.

11. Ando G, Morabito G, de Gregorio C, et al. Age, glomerular filtration rate, ejection fraction, and the AGEF score predict contrast-induced nephropathy in patients with acute myocardial infarction undergoing primary percutaneous coronary intervention. Catheter Cardiovasc Interv 2013;82(6):878–85.

12. Gurm HS, Seth M, Kooiman J, et al. A novel tool for reliable and accurate prediction of renal complications in patients undergoing percutaneous coronary intervention. J Am Coll Cardiol 2013;61(22):2242–8.

13. Maioli M, Toso A, Gallopin M, et al. Preprocedural score for risk of contrast-induced nephropathy in elective coronary angiography and intervention. J Cardiovasc Med 2010;11(6):444–9.

14. Brown JR, DeVries JT, Piper WD, et al. Serious renal dysfunction after percutaneous coronary interventions can be predicted. Am Heart J 2008;155(2):260–6.

15. Mehran R, Aymong ED, Nikolsky E, et al. A simple risk score for prediction of contrast-induced nephropathy after percutaneous coronary intervention: development and initial validation. J Am Coll Cardiol 2004;44(7):1393–9.

16. Iakovou I, Dangas G, Mehran R, et al. Impact of gender on the incidence and outcome of contrast-induced nephropathy after percutaneous coronary intervention. J Invasive Cardiol 2003;15(1):18–22.

17. Gruberg L, Mehran R, Dangas G, et al. Acute renal failure requiring dialysis after percutaneous coronary interventions. Catheter Cardiovasc Interv 2001;52(4):409–16.

18. McCullough PA, Wolyn R, Rocher LL, et al. Acute renal failure after coronary intervention: incidence, risk factors, and relationship to mortality. Am J Med 1997;103(5):368–75.

19. Tajti P, Karatasakis A, Danek BA, et al. In-Hospital Outcomes of Chronic Total Occlusion Percutaneous Coronary Intervention in Patients With Chronic Kidney Disease. J Invasive Cardiol 2018;30(11):E113–21.

20. Kroll RG, Yelavarthy P, Menees DS, et al. Predicting Contrast-Induced Renal Complications. Interv Cardiol Clin 2020;9(3):321–33.

21. Gupta RK, Bang TJ. Prevention of Contrast-Induced Nephropathy (CIN) in Interventional Radiology Practice. Semin Intervent Radiol 2010;27(4):348–59.

22. Tsai TT, Patel UD, Chang TI, et al. Contemporary incidence, predictors, and outcomes of acute kidney injury in patients undergoing percutaneous coronary interventions: insights from the NCDR Cath-PCI registry. JACC Cardiovasc Interv 2014;7(1):1–9.

23. Gurm HS, Smith D, Share D, et al. Impact of automated contrast injector systems on contrast use and contrast-associated complications in patients undergoing percutaneous coronary interventions. JACC Cardiovasc Interv 2013;6(4):399–405.

24. Rihal CS, Textor SC, Grill DE, et al. Incidence and prognostic importance of acute renal failure after percutaneous coronary intervention. Circulation 2002;105(19):2259–64.

25. Parfrey PS, Griffiths SM, Barrett BJ, et al. Contrast material-induced renal failure in patients with diabetes mellitus, renal insufficiency, or both. A prospective controlled study. N Engl J Med 1989;320(3):143–9.

26. Heyman SN, Rosenberger C, Rosen S, et al. Why is diabetes mellitus a risk factor for contrast-induced nephropathy? BioMed Res Int 2013;2013:123589.

27. Turcot DB, Kiernan FJ, McKay RG, et al. Acute hyperglycemia: implications for contrast-induced nephropathy during cardiac catheterization. Diabetes Care. Feb 2004;27(2):620–1.

28. Marenzi G, Lauri G, Assanelli E, et al. Contrast-induced nephropathy in patients undergoing primary angioplasty for acute myocardial infarction. J Am Coll Cardiol 2004;44(9):1780–5.

29. Chen H, Yu X, Ma L. Risk factors of contrast-induced nephropathy in patients with STEMI and pump failure undergoing percutaneous coronary intervention. Exp Ther Med 2021;21(2):140.

30. Dangas G, Iakovou I, Nikolsky E, et al. Contrast-induced nephropathy after percutaneous coronary interventions in relation to chronic kidney disease and hemodynamic variables. Am J Cardiol 2005;95(1):13–9.

31. Lindsay J, Canos DA, Apple S, et al. Causes of acute renal dysfunction after percutaneous coronary intervention and comparison of late mortality rates with postprocedure rise of creatine kinase-

MB versus rise of serum creatinine. Am J Cardiol 2004;94(6):786–9.

32. Bartholomew BA, Harjai KJ, Dukkipati S, et al. Impact of nephropathy after percutaneous coronary intervention and a method for risk stratification. Am J Cardiol 2004;93(12):1515–9.

33. Brar SS, Aharonian V, Mansukhani P, et al. Haemodynamic-guided fluid administration for the prevention of contrast-induced acute kidney injury: the POSEIDON randomised controlled trial. Lancet 2014;383(9931):1814–23.

34. Nikolsky E, Mehran R, Lasic Z, et al. Low hematocrit predicts contrast-induced nephropathy after percutaneous coronary interventions. Kidney Int 2005;67(2):706–13.

35. Ohno Y, Maekawa Y, Miyata H, et al. Impact of periprocedural bleeding on incidence of contrast-induced acute kidney injury in patients treated with percutaneous coronary intervention. J Am Coll Cardiol 2013;62(14):1260–6.

36. Brener MI, Bush A, Miller JM, et al. Influence of radial versus femoral access site on coronary angiography and intervention outcomes: A systematic review and meta-analysis. Catheter Cardiovasc Interv 2017;90(7):1093–104.

37. Rao SV, Hess CN, Barham B, et al. A registry-based randomized trial comparing radial and femoral approaches in women undergoing percutaneous coronary intervention: the SAFE-PCI for Women (Study of Access Site for Enhancement of PCI for Women) trial. JACC Cardiovasc Interv 2014;7(8):857–67.

38. Sutton NR, Seth M, Lingam N, et al. Radial Access Use for Percutaneous Coronary Intervention in Dialysis Patients. Circ Cardiovasc Interv 2020;13(1):e008418.

39. Kooiman J, Seth M, Dixon S, et al. Risk of acute kidney injury after percutaneous coronary interventions using radial versus femoral vascular access: insights from the Blue Cross Blue Shield of Michigan Cardiovascular Consortium. Circ Cardiovasc Interv 2014;7(2):190–8.

40. Ando G, Cortese B, Russo F, et al. Acute Kidney Injury After Radial or Femoral Access for Invasive Acute Coronary Syndrome Management: AKI-MATRIX. J Am Coll Cardiol 2017. https://doi.org/10.1016/j.jacc.2017.02.070.

41. Seeliger E, Sendeski M, Rihal CS, et al. Contrast-induced kidney injury: mechanisms, risk factors, and prevention. Eur Heart J 2012;33(16):2007–15.

42. Kawatani Y, Kurobe H, Nakamura Y, et al. The ratio of contrast medium volume to estimated glomerular filtration rate as a predictor of contrast-induced nephropathy after endovascular aortic repair. J Med Invest 2018;65(12):116–21.

43. Nyman U, Bjork J, Aspelin P, et al. Contrast medium dose-to-GFR ratio: a measure of systemic exposure to predict contrast-induced nephropathy after percutaneous coronary intervention. Acta Radiol 2008;49(6):658–67.

44. Ando G, de Gregorio C, Morabito G, et al. Renal function-adjusted contrast volume redefines the baseline estimation of contrast-induced acute kidney injury risk in patients undergoing primary percutaneous coronary intervention. Circ Cardiovasc Interv 2014;7(4):465–72.

45. Tan N, Liu Y, Chen JY, et al. Use of the contrast volume or grams of iodine-to-creatinine clearance ratio to predict mortality after percutaneous coronary intervention. Am Heart J 2013;165(4):600–8.

46. Gurm HS, Dixon SR, Smith DE, et al. Renal function-based contrast dosing to define safe limits of radiographic contrast media in patients undergoing percutaneous coronary interventions. J Am Coll Cardiol 2011;58(9):907–14.

47. Liu Y, Liu YH, Chen JY, et al. Safe contrast volumes for preventing contrast-induced nephropathy in elderly patients with relatively normal renal function during percutaneous coronary intervention. Medicine (Baltim) 2015;94(12):e615.

48. Laskey WK, Jenkins C, Selzer F, et al. Volume-to-creatinine clearance ratio: a pharmacokinetically based risk factor for prediction of early creatinine increase after percutaneous coronary intervention. J Am Coll Cardiol 2007;50(7):584–90.

49. Cigarroa RG, Lange RA, Williams RH, et al. Dosing of contrast material to prevent contrast nephropathy in patients with renal disease. Am J Med 1989;86(6 Pt 1):649–52.

50. Brown JR, Robb JF, Block CA, et al. Does safe dosing of iodinated contrast prevent contrast-induced acute kidney injury? Circ Cardiovasc Interv 2010;3(4):346–50.

51. Marenzi G, Assanelli E, Campodonico J, et al. Contrast volume during primary percutaneous coronary intervention and subsequent contrast-induced nephropathy and mortality. Ann Intern Med 2009;150(3):170–7.

52. Gurm HS, Seth M, Dixon SR, et al. Contemporary use of and outcomes associated with ultra-low contrast volume in patients undergoing percutaneous coronary interventions. Catheter Cardiovasc Interv 2019;93(2):222–30.

53. Rahim HM, Flattery E, Gkargkoulas F, et al. Ultra-low-contrast angiography in patients with advanced chronic kidney disease and previous coronary artery bypass surgery. Coron Artery Dis 2019;30(5):346–51.

54. Hatem R, Finn MT, Riley RF, et al. Zero contrast retrograde chronic total occlusions percutaneous coronary intervention: a case series. Eur Heart J Case Rep 2018;2(2):1–5.

55. Karimi Galougahi K, Mintz GS, Karmpaliotis D, et al. Zero-contrast percutaneous coronary intervention on calcified lesions facilitated by rotational atherectomy. Catheter Cardiovasc Interv 2017;90(4):E85–9.

56. Karimi Galougahi K, Zalewski A, Leon MB, et al. Optical coherence tomography-guided percutaneous coronary intervention in pre-terminal chronic kidney disease with no radio-contrast administration. Eur Heart J 2016;37(13):1059.

57. Cho KJ. Carbon Dioxide Angiography: Scientific Principles and Practice. Vasc Specialist Int 2015; 31(3):67–80.

58. De Lima JJ, Gowdak LH, de Paula FJ, et al. Coronary Artery Disease Assessment and Intervention in Renal Transplant Patients: Analysis from the KiHeart Cohort. Transplantation 2016;100(7):1580–7.

59. De Lima JJ, Gowdak LH, de Paula FJ, et al. Treatment of coronary artery disease in hemodialysis patients evaluated for transplant-a registry study. Transplantation 2010;89(7):845–50.

60. Patel RK, Mark PB, Johnston N, et al. Prognostic value of cardiovascular screening in potential renal transplant recipients: a single-center prospective observational study. Am J Transplant 2008;8(8): 1673–83.

61. Jones DG, Taylor AM, Enkiri SA, et al. Extent and severity of coronary disease and mortality in patients with end-stage renal failure evaluated for renal transplantation. Am J Transplant 2009;9(8): 1846–52.

62. Mehta RL, Kellum JA, Shah SV, et al. Acute Kidney Injury Network: report of an initiative to improve outcomes in acute kidney injury. Crit Care 2007; 11(2):R31.

63. Bellomo R, Kellum JA, Ronco C. Defining and classifying acute renal failure: from advocacy to consensus and validation of the RIFLE criteria. Intensive Care Med 2007;33(3):409–13.

64. Capodanno D, Ministeri M, Cumbo S, et al. Volume-to-creatinine clearance ratio in patients undergoing coronary angiography with or without percutaneous coronary intervention: implications of varying definitions of contrast-induced nephropathy. Catheter Cardiovasc Interv 2014;83(6):907–12.

65. Ohman EM, Granger CB, Harrington RA, et al. Risk stratification and therapeutic decision making in acute coronary syndromes. JAMA 2000;284(7):876–8.

66. Freeman RV, O'Donnell M, Share D, et al. Nephropathy requiring dialysis after percutaneous coronary intervention and the critical role of an adjusted contrast dose. Am J Cardiol 2002;90(10): 1068–73.

67. Aykan AC, Gul I, Gokdeniz T, et al. Is coronary artery disease complexity valuable in the prediction of contrast induced nephropathy besides Mehran risk score, in patients with ST elevation myocardial infarction treated with primary percutaneous coronary intervention? Heart Lung Circ 2013;22(10):836–43.

68. Raposeiras-Roubin S, Abu-Assi E, Ocaranza-Sanchez R, et al. Dosing of iodinated contrast volume: a new simple algorithm to stratify the risk of contrast-induced nephropathy in patients with acute coronary syndrome. Catheter Cardiovasc Interv 2013;82(6):888–97.

69. Sgura FA, Bertelli L, Monopoli D, et al. Mehran contrast-induced nephropathy risk score predicts short- and long-term clinical outcomes in patients with ST-elevation-myocardial infarction. Circ Cardiovasc Interv 2010;3(5):491–8.

70. Mehran R, Owen R, Chiarito M, et al. A contemporary simple risk score for prediction of contrast-associated acute kidney injury after percutaneous coronary intervention: derivation and validation from an observational registry. Lancet 2021;398(10315):1974–83.

71. Skelding KA, Best PJ, Bartholomew BA, et al. Validation of a predictive risk score for radiocontrast-induced nephropathy following percutaneous coronary intervention. J Invasive Cardiol 2007; 19(5):229–33.

72. Gu G, Yuan X, Zhou Y, et al. Elevated high-sensitivity C-reactive protein combined with procalcitonin predicts high risk of contrast-induced nephropathy after percutaneous coronary intervention. BMC Cardiovasc Disord 2019;19(1):152.

73. Reyes LF, Severiche-Bueno DF, Bustamante CA, et al. Serum levels of neutrophil Gelatinase associated Lipocalin (NGAL) predicts hemodialysis after coronary angiography in high risk patients with acute coronary syndrome. BMC Nephrol 2020; 21(1):143.

74. Zhang JY, Wang Q, Wang RT, et al. Increased urinary adiponectin level is associated with contrast-induced nephropathy in patients undergoing elective percutaneous coronary intervention. BMC Cardiovasc Disord 2019;19(1):160.

75. Jaroszynski A, Zaborowski T, Gluszek S, et al. Heat Shock Protein 27 Is an Emerging Predictor of Contrast-Induced Acute Kidney Injury on Patients Subjected to Percutaneous Coronary Interventions. Cells 2021;10(3).

76. Mohebi R, van Kimmenade R, McCarthy C, et al. A Biomarker-Enhanced Model for Prediction of Acute Kidney Injury and Cardiovascular Risk Following Angiographic Procedures: CASA-BLANCA AKI Prediction Substudy. J Am Heart Assoc 2022;11(10):e025729.

77. Yuan N, Zhang J, Khaki R, et al. Implementation of an Electronic Health Records-Based Safe Contrast Limit for Preventing Contrast-Associated Acute Kidney Injury After Percutaneous Coronary Intervention. Circ Cardiovasc Qual Outcomes 2023;16(1): e009235.

78. Kulkarni H, Amin AP. Artificial intelligence in percutaneous coronary intervention: improved risk prediction of PCI-related complications using an artificial neural network. BMJ Innovations 2021;7(3):564–79.

79. Li D, Jiang H, Yang X, et al. An Online Preprocedural Nomogram for the Prediction of

Contrast-Associated Acute Kidney Injury in Patients Undergoing Coronary Angiography. Front Med 2022;9:839856.

80. Barbieri L, Verdoia M, Marino P, et al. Contrast volume to creatinine clearance ratio for the prediction of contrast-induced nephropathy in patients undergoing coronary angiography or percutaneous intervention. Eur J Prev Cardiol 2016;23(9):931–7.

81. Victor SM, Gnanaraj A, Suma V, et al. Risk scoring system to predict contrast induced nephropathy following percutaneous coronary intervention. Indian Heart J 2014;66(5):517–24.

82. Tziakas D, Chalikias G, Stakos D, et al. Development of an easily applicable risk score model for contrast-induced nephropathy prediction after percutaneous coronary intervention: a novel approach tailored to current practice. Int J Cardiol 2013;163(1):46–55.

83. Chong E, Shen L, Poh KK, et al. Risk scoring system for prediction of contrast-induced nephropathy in patients with pre-existing renal impairment undergoing percutaneous coronary intervention. Singapore Med J 2012;53(3):164–9.

84. Tan N, Liu Y, Zhou YL, et al. Contrast medium volume to creatinine clearance ratio: a predictor of contrast-induced nephropathy in the first 72 hours following percutaneous coronary intervention. Catheter Cardiovasc Interv 2012;79(1):70–5.

85. Fu NK, Yang SC, Chen YL, et al. [Risk factors and scoring system in the prediction of contrast induced nephropathy in patients undergoing percutaneous coronary intervention]. Zhonghua Yixue Zazhi 2012;92(8):551–4.

86. Ghani AA, Tohamy KY. Risk score for contrast induced nephropathy following percutaneous coronary intervention. Saudi J Kidney Dis Transpl 2009; 20(2):240–5.

Hydration to Prevent Contrast-Associated Acute Kidney Injury in Patients Undergoing Cardiac Angiography

Richard Solomon, MD

KEYWORDS

• Hydration • Water • Saline • Acute kidney injury • Contrast medium • Cardiac • Angiography

---

KEY POINTS

- Giving of water or fluid as *treatment* is well grounded in medical practice.
- Fluids are appropriate and should be given to patients with symptoms and signs directly related to loss of body fluid, for example, bleeding, severe dehydration, diarrhea, and so on.
- The use of fluids to *prevent* symptoms and signs associated with a particular disease process is far less grounded.
- Focusing on patients undergoing cardiac catheterization and the evidence that hydration can prevent or at least minimize the risk of contrast-associated acute kidney injury (CA-AKI).
- CA-AKI is used in favor of contrast-induced acute kidney injury or contrast-induced nephropathy because these patients are also exposed to many other insults such as hemodynamic alterations (ischemia) and atheroembolic disease in addition to a nephrotoxin (contrast media).

INTRODUCTION

The current guideline from the American College of Cardiology/American Heart Association recommend use of "hydration" for prophylaxis for acute kidney injury (AKI) following the administration of contrast in the catheterization laboratory particularly in high- risk patients but give no guidance on type of fluid, how much to give, and when to give it.[1] The word "hydration" means the process of making your body absorb water or other liquid. The giving of water or fluid as *treatment* is well grounded in medical practice. Common sense dictates that fluids are appropriate and should be given to patients with symptoms and signs directly related to loss of body fluid, for example, bleeding, severe dehydration, diarrhea, and so on. However, the use of fluids to *prevent* symptoms and signs associated with a particular disease process is far less grounded. In this chapter, the author presents the evidence favoring a *preventative* effect of fluid administration and focus on patients undergoing cardiac catheterization and the evidence that hydration can prevent or at least minimize the risk of contrast-associated acute kidney injury (CA-AKI). The term "contrast-associated acute kidney injury" is used in favor of contrast-induced acute kidney injury (CI-AKI) or contrast-induced nephropathy (CIN) because these patients are also exposed to many other insults such as hemodynamic alterations (ischemia), and atheroembolic disease in addition to a nephrotoxin (contrast media). All these insults may contribute to an acute impairment of kidney function.

WHAT DOES HYDRATION DO PHYSIOLOGICALLY?

All fluids are not alike, and this is a problem with the general recommendation to hydrate. In the context of mitigating kidney injury in patients

---

Larner College of Medicine, University of Vermont, Burlington, VT 05401, USA
E-mail address: Richard.Solomon@uvmhealth.org

Intervent Cardiol Clin 12 (2023) 515–524
https://doi.org/10.1016/j.iccl.2023.06.009

undergoing cardiac catheterization procedures, oral water and intravenous (IV) half normal sodium chloride, isotonic sodium chloride, and isotonic sodium bicarbonate have all been studied in clinical trials. In this article the author briefly reviews what administration of any of these fluids does physiologically (Table 1).

Oral Water

Ingestion of water (without solute) rapidly dilutes the solute level (osmolality) throughout body fluids. Serum osmolality is the main determinant of vasopressin levels. As a result of lowering serum osmolality and vasopressin levels, aquaporin 2 channels are rapidly recycled into the cytoplasm of renal collecting tubule cells, greatly reducing the transport of water out of the lumen of the collecting tubule. As a result, urine osmolality drops and urine output increases. This increase in urine output occurs without a change in glomerular filtration rate (GFR) or function of earlier segments of the nephron. Because vasopressin is also responsible for the insertion of urea reabsorbing transporters, the excretion of urea increases with an oral water load.[2]

Oral water ingestion is not an efficient way to expand intravascular volume because only 1/12 of the absorbed water will remain in the intravascular compartment. A simple math exercise shows how impractical and potentially dangerous intravascular volume expansion with water can be. To achieve a 10% expansion of intravascular volume (4L→ 4.4 L) would require administration of 4.8 L of water (1/12 staying in the intravascular compartment); this would dilute serum osmolality and sodium by 10% (280→252 and 140→126, respectively). Not safe!

Intravenous Isotonic Saline

This is the standard of care when it comes to fluids for expansion of intravascular volume.

With isotonic saline, one-fourth of the administered fluid remains in the intravascular space. Following the example earlier, to expand the intravascular space by 10% (400 mL) requires 1.2 L of fluid and does not alter serum osmolality or sodium unless very large amounts are administered (because isotonic saline has an osmolality of 300 and sodium of 155, both higher than normal). The intravascular volume expansion that can be achieved will likely have secondary physiologic consequences. Cardiac output may increase as a result of an increase in preload (Starling curve), resulting in an increase in kidney perfusion. Volume-sensing hormonal and neurologic systems may downregulate via baroreceptor inhibition, for example, a decrease in the activity of the renin-angiotensin system and sympathetic nervous system and an increase in natriuretic peptide secretion. Serum oncotic pressure may decrease; this may have downstream effects on kidney handling of sodium, ultimately resulting in a natriuresis and an increase in urine output. These systems are designed to maintain homeostasis. Load the body with salt and water, and normal physiologic processes will be activated to get rid of that load.

The time frame of these changes may be important when we consider fluids as therapy. With water loads, the effects occur within minutes, and maximum increases in urine output and reduction in urine osmolality occur within an hour with return to preload conditions within 4 to 6 hours. In the case of isotonic saline, the adaptions are much slower and return to baseline may take days. Isotonic saline provides a more sustained increase in intravascular volume (and its downstream physiologic effects) for that reason.

Intravenous Isotonic Sodium Bicarbonate

The major difference between isotonic sodium chloride and sodium bicarbonate is the effect

Table 1
Physiologic effects of hydration solutions and the expected effect on the kidney (in bold)

	Oral Water	0.9% Saline	Isotonic Bicarb	0.45% Saline
Intravascular volume	→	↑↑	↑↑	↑
Cardiac output	→	↑↑	↑↑	↑
Renal blood flow	→	↑↑	↑↑	↑
RAAS, SNS	→	↓↓	↓↓	↓
Natriuretic peptides	→	↑↑	↑↑	↑
Natriuresis	→	↑↑	↑↑	↑
Vasopressin	↓↓↓	↓	↓	↓↓
Urine output	↑↑↑	↑	↑	↑↑

of chloride. When many liters of fluid are to be administered, isotonic sodium chloride can lead to hyperchloremia, which has been associated with a decrease in renal perfusion. This does not occur with isotonic sodium bicarbonate or any other "balanced salt solution" for that matter. In addition, isotonic sodium bicarbonate raises intravascular pH slightly, whereas isotonic saline does the opposite. The extent to which systemic acid-base changes are relevant to kidney function and/or protection from kidney injury is unclear.[3]

Intravenous 0.45% Saline
One can consider this a mix of water and isotonic saline. Less of this fluid will be retained in the intravascular space, resulting in less potential impact on cardiac output and those neurohumoral systems noted earlier. Urine output should increase because the hypotonicity of the administered fluid should suppress vasopressin.

Clinical Trial Data
The fluids described earlier have all been studied in clinical trials (observational and prospective randomized). The primary outcome has been acute kidney injury, variously defined as some combination of an absolute increase in serum creatinine of 0.3 mg/dL, 0.5 mg/dL, or 1.0 mg/dL within a few days of the cardiac catheterization or a percentage increase in serum creatinine of 25% or 50% in that same period of time. Besides this primary outcome, the clinical trial data provide insights into how much fluid is necessary for achieving the primary outcome, when it was started and stopped, what rate it is given at, and what patients benefitted the most. Finally, long-term outcomes such as progression of chronic kidney disease, need for dialysis, and mortality have been evaluated in some trials.

Before diving into the trial data, we need some reference points. To start with, how often does AKI, the primary outcome, occur following coronary angiography? The National Cardiovascular Data Registry (NCDR) is probably the best source of information. The NCDR defines postpercutaneous coronary intervention AKI (PCI-AKI) as an increase in serum creatinine of 0.3 mg/dL or 50% or new onset of dialysis occurring during the hospitalization following the PCI. Based on that definition, post-PCI-AKI occurs in ~14% of the total population, with rates up to 50% in some high-risk populations.[4] These data come from analyses of the 2012 reporting of more than 650,000 patients, which corresponds to the time frame of many of the studies discussed later. The lowest decile of hospitals in

the report had an AKI rate of 5.7%. When a clinical trial reports a rate much less than this in the "control" group, one should be very concerned that they have chosen a very low-risk group to study, for example, diagnostic studies with low-contrast volumes or inclusion of IV contrast for computed tomography scans. Although there may be statistical significance in the trial, the clinical relevance should be questioned.

Hydration Versus No-Hydration
In 1981, Eisenberg observed no cases of CA-AKI (>1 mg/dL increase in creatinine at 24 hours) in patients undergoing a variety of arteriograms with *high-osmolar* contrast media when given 550 mL/h of 0.9% NaCl during angiography.[5] The infusion of 0.9% saline was expected to replace the loss of fluid and electrolytes resulting from the osmotic diuresis induced by the contrast. Thus, it was to prevent dehydration and volume depletion. Although use of high-osmolar contrast was discontinued a decade later, hydration remained the standard of care for patients exposed to contrast.

A randomized trial with a no-hydration control group was not published until 2008, such was the belief in the advantages of hydration. A trial that included high-risk patients by Chen and colleagues compared no-hydration with 0.45% NaCl for 28 hours, beginning 4 hours before angiography and for 24 hours after angiography.[6] An advantage of hydration was seen only in patients with chronic kidney disease (CA-AKI 34% no hydration vs 21% hydration). Three subsequent trials studied ST-elevation myocardial infarction (STEMI) patients. Maioli studied 300 patients who were randomized to no-hydration versus 0.9% NaCl at 1 mL/kg/h for 12 hours after primary PCI. The incidence of CA-AKI was 27% versus 22%, respectively (not significant). However, a third group that received IV 0.9% NaCl before *and* after PCI had an incidence of 12%.[7] Two additional trials in patients with STEMI confirmed that IV 0.9% NaCl was superior to no-hydration in preventing CA-AKI. Rates of CA-AKI were significantly reduced by giving 0.9% NaCl at 1 mL/kg/h for 12 to 24 hours following primary PCI.[8,9] Finally, a recent trial in 401 non-ST-elevation myocardial infarction patients also found hydration (with 0.9% saline 1 mL/kg/h given for 3–12 hours before and 24 hours after contrast exposure) superior to no-hydration (CA-AKI 7.1% vs 14.1%, respectively).[10] A subsequent meta-analysis of ~1000 patients found that hydration significantly reduced the risk of CA-AKI (risk ratio 0.64 in those with estimated GFR [eGFR] 30–60 mL/min) as well as need for renal replacement and mortality.[11]

More recently, a trial in patients receiving both IV and intra-arterial contrast found no benefit to hydration. The trial was appropriately named AMACING (A MAstricht Contrast-Induced Nephropathy Guideline). All patients had eGFR between 30 and 60 mL/min. The hydration (isotonic saline before and after, dose dependent on medical grounds) and no-hydration groups had rates of CA-AKI of 2.6% and 2.7%, respectively (~4% for intraarterial contrast).[12] These patients were clearly low risk; only 15% underwent an intervention, and the average amount of contrast administered was 90 mL. They received much smaller volumes of contrast than typically used in a coronary intervention, and only a single creatinine was obtained up to 6 days postprocedure, raising the concern that some CA-AKI could have been missed. There was also substantial missing data (9%) that could have influenced the results. A meta-analysis specifically looking at factors that influenced the efficacy of hydration strategies found them to be effective only when contrast volume was greater than 100 mL.[13]

Oral Water

There are many observational and randomized trials that have examined the effect of oral hydration with water on the outcome of CA-AKI. These trials have reported equivalency between oral and IV hydration (see meta-analyses[14,15]) but are limited by small size, mixture of IV and oral fluid in the "oral" group, and/or lack of prespecified amount of oral fluid to be given. Prospective randomized trials comparing a specific amount and timing of oral hydration versus IV saline in patients undergoing coronary angiography found equivalency between oral water (~1000 mL) and similar amounts of IV saline.[16,17] The total number of patients in these trials is ~1000. Not all patients had impaired kidney function, and rates of CA-AKI in the IV saline groups ranged from 5% to 22%. A 2021 observational trial in 754 STEMI patients found that there was a declining incidence of CA-AKI when patients drank more than 15.7 mL/kg over the 24 hours following primary PCI.[18] Although these trials are provocative in that they challenge our understanding of a mechanism of action for hydration prevention of kidney injury, they are insufficient to recommend replacing IV fluid with oral fluid for high-risk patients. They also raise a confounding issue for all the trials in which control over oral intake of fluid was not protocolized.

Intravenous Saline

A single randomized trial in 2002 compared 0.9% versus 0.45% saline in 1620 patients undergoing coronary angiography and found superiority to 0.9% saline (CA-AKI 0.7% vs 2.0%) using a definition of CA-AKI of greater than 0.5 mg/dL increase within 48 hours. However, similar to the AMACING trial, these were not high-risk patients. Baseline eGFR was 84 mL/min. Subgroup analyses showed that only women, patients with diabetes, and those receiving greater than 250 mL of contrast did better with 0.9%,[19] but there was no advantage in those with mild chronic kidney disease. A trial by Marron compared 2000 mL of 0.9% saline with a similar volume of 0.45% saline administered over 24 hours, beginning 12 hours before coronary angiography and continuing for 12 hours afterward in 71 patients (25% with chronic kidney disease).[20] There were no differences in the incidence of CA-AKI (13.5% and 11.7%, respectively) or in urine output over the 24 hours. Thus, the evidence favoring isotonic over hypotonic fluid is not compelling because of the paucity of high-risk patients.

Intravenous Sodium Bicarbonate

Many randomized trials have been conducted comparing isotonic saline with isotonic bicarbonate. The rationale for the use of bicarbonate was based on an initial trial by Merten[21] and the hypothesis that alkalinization inhibited the generation of free radicals thought to play a role in the pathogenesis of CA-AKI (see chapter 3). The PRESERVE trial[22] compared more than 5000 patients undergoing coronary angiography (diagnostic and intervention) and compared isotonic saline and isotonic bicarbonate. The primary endpoint was a composite of death, the need for dialysis, or a persistent increase in serum creatinine of at least 50% postcontrast media. More than half of the patients had an eGFR of 15 to 44.9 mL/min/1.73 m^2, and 80% were diabetic, which puts the majority at moderate to high risk for CA-AKI. It found no significant difference between the groups in the primary endpoint (4.4% sodium bicarbonate vs 4.7% isotonic saline; $P = .6$) or the development of CA-AKI (9.5% sodium bicarbonate vs 8.3% isotonic saline; $P = .13$). In addition, instead of finding the preventive benefit of sodium bicarbonate, use of it was associated with disadvantages, such as its expense and the potential for error from compounding it. These data can be interpreted as supporting the use of sodium chloride.

How much fluid is recommended and when should it be given?

In the absence of a clear mechanism of action for decreasing the incidence of CA-AKI, the following is my personal recommendation.

- More fluid is better than less (Table 2)
- Fluid should be given before as well as after exposure to insult

What is the evidence?

First, 3 trials of CA-AKI prophylaxis used hemodynamic monitoring or assessment of body fluid status to determine the amount of fluid to be given. One approach used left ventricular end-diastolic pressure (LVEDP) to determine the rate at which 0.9% saline was to be administered and compared it with standard of care.[23] All patients received a 3 mL/kg bolus during the hour preprocedure, 1.5 mL/kg/h during the procedure, and then a variable amount (1–5 mL/kg/h) for 4 hours postprocedure. As shown in Table 2, the rates of CA-AKI decreased in a stepwise fashion as the volume of fluid administered increased. There were no differences in 30-day or 6-month adverse events between the LVEDP and standard-of-care approach. A small trial repeated this protocol but did not find a difference in CA-AKI.[24] However, they provided IV 0.9% saline for 12 hours before and after angiography in the control group and did not report that the LVEDP-guided group received more IV fluid.

A second hemodynamic-guided approach used central venous pressure (CVP) measurements during the procedure and adjusted the rate of fluid delivery according to the CVP readings. Those with lower CVP received more fluid.[25] As shown in Table 2, more fluid was associated with a lower incidence of CA-AKI.

A third trial used bioimpedance vector analysis (BIVA) to determine the rate of fluid administration. Those with "optimal" preangiography values received 1 mL/kg/h of 0.9% saline for 12 hours before and after the procedure. Those with low BIVA values received 2 mL/kg/h for 12 hours before and after the procedure.[26]

These 3 trials favor the administration of more fluid for prophylaxis of CA-AKI, and the use of prefluid administration monitoring allowed greater amounts of fluid to be administered safely. One could raise the argument that patients with preangiography low LVEDP, CVP, or BIVA are somehow less likely to develop CA-AKI and that the lower incidence of CA-AKI in those groups is independent of the amount of fluid administered. However, a compelling mechanism by which that might occur is unclear. These trials also excluded or adjusted the rate of hydration based on a history of heart failure. An observational study in 1307 patients with heart failure undergoing cardiac angiography found that increasing hydration volume was associated with worse CA-AKI. However, there were many other CA-AKI risk factors in those who received the most fluid that might have biased the results despite attempts to adjust statistically.[27]

More recently the data from the PRESERVE trial have been analyzed to see if the amount of IV fluid affected the incidence of CA-AKI.[28] The amount of fluid administered was determined at each site and was not protocolized. The 4471 patients who had sufficient data were divided into quartiles based on the amount of fluid administered. There was no difference in the rate of CA-AKI across the quartiles that were not necessarily matched for risk factors for CA-AKI. These post-hoc data therefore do not provide any guidance for how much fluid to administer.

Timing of Fluid Administration

The management of patients with acute coronary syndromes has increasingly been driven to minimizing in-patient care. Most elective coronary angiograms and interventions encourage discharge from the hospital within 24 hours, and even STEMI patients are spending less time in the hospital; this complicates not only diagnosing CA-AKI but prescribing fluid for prophylaxis. A few, small randomized trials compared giving IV fluid for up to 12 hours preangiography with either an equal volume given over 6 hours or as a bolus just before angiography.[29,30] Both trials showed that the longer duration was more favorable. These results do support a

Table 2
Relationship between amount of fluid administered and incidence of contrast-associated acute kidney injury

Group	Amount of 0.9% Saline Administered (mL)	Incidence of CA-AKI[a] (%)
1 LVEDP	448–874	17
2 LVEDP	874–1512	11
3 LVEDP	1512–3055	6
1 CVP	500–1000	38
2 CVP	1000–1500	31
3 CVP	>1500	8
1 BIVA	961–1680	11
2 BIVA	2522–3600	5

[a] CA-AKI defined as >0.3 mg/dL increase in creatinine in LVEDP and BIVA trials; CA-AKI defined as >25% or >0.5 mg/dL increase in creatinine in CVP trial.

Data abstracted from: LVEDP (22), CVP (24) and BIVA (25) trials.

mechanism of action of fluid administration that requires some time to activate.

A recent trial in 508 STEMI patients found that the incidence of CA-AKI between a group randomized to receive hydration for 24 hours postprocedure versus 12 hours postprocedure but with the same total fluid intake was the same (~9%).[31] The higher fluid rate in the latter group was achieved with the use of IV furosemide to prevent possible volume overload.

Urine Output

The benefits associated with giving more fluid and starting "hydration" earlier are also associated with stimulating an increase in urine output. Indeed, several trials found an inverse correlation between the amount of urine produced and the incidence of CA-AKI[32,33] (Fig. 1). The mechanisms behind the potential beneficial effects of a large urine output on CA-AKI are reviewed elsewhere.[34] The focus on urine output has led to several attempts to stimulate an increase in urine output specifically to reduce the incidence of CA-AKI.

Forced Diuresis

Multiple randomized trials have randomized patients to hydration versus hydration with furosemide. The doses of furosemide were ~1 mg/kg administered just before angiography. These trials all found worse outcomes in the furosemide group.[35–38] Notably, attempts to maintain a stable weight were unsuccessful, and most patients lost weight by 24 hours; this raises the possibility that activation of sodium-retaining mechanisms within the kidney, decreases in cardiac output and renal blood flow, and other physiologic effects of volume depletion all contributed to the negative results. Subsequently, more recent trials used smaller doses of furosemide (~0.25 mg/kg) and carefully replaced urine losses. These trials tended to show a benefit of additional furosemide.[39,40] In clinical practice, ensuring replacement of urine losses is not easy and requires significant personnel resources.

Forced Matched Diuresis

The RenalGuard device weighs urine output collected in a Foley bag (drop by drop) and instantaneously infuses an equal volume of 0.9% saline to prevent any net volume loss. Randomized trials comparing the use of this device versus standard-of-care IV fluid administration (usually 1 mL/kg/h) both before and after angiography have shown a benefit of this approach.[41–47] Subjects in the RenalGuard group receive 250 mL of IV 0.9% saline and 0.25 mg/kg of furosemide starting about 1 hour before angiography. At the start of angiography, urine output is usually greater than 300 mL/h and continues to increase to 500 to 600 mL/h during the procedure and gradually decreases over the next 6 hours when therapy is stopped. This therapy has been used in patients undergoing PCI, transcatheter aortic valve replacement (TAVR), and coronary artery bypass graft (CABG), with consistent results showing a reduction in the incidence of AKI.[47] A meta-analysis of these trials was published in 2021.[47] Finally, a trial comparing forced matched diuresis with LVEDP-guided hydration therapy found the former superior in prevention of CA-AKI and with lower rates of pulmonary embolus and 1-month major adverse cardiac events. There was more hypokalemia, however.[48] The therapy is currently approved in Europe but

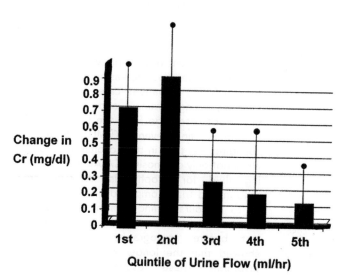

Fig. 1. Change in postcontrast creatinine by amount of urine output in first 24 hours. (*From* Prince study.[32])

not in the United States pending Food and Drug Administration approval. Its major downside is the need for a Foley catheter. The upside is that it is easily adapted to same day discharge of uncomplicated procedures. Use of a nonautomated forced matched diuresis regime was recently reported to be superior to standard-of-care IV hydration (1–1.5 mL/kg/h saline 12 hours before and after PCI).[49] This, however, required staff to record output every 5 minutes and replace accordingly.

SUMMARY

Administration of isotonic fluid before, during, and after exposure to intraarterial contrast in patients at risk of developing CA-AKI reduces that risk. The mechanism of benefit is unclear. An increase in urine output seems to be an important component. The evidence suggests that an increase in urine output and reduction in CA-AKI can be achieved with oral water, 0.45% or 0.9% saline, although most of the studies used 0.9% saline. A recent network meta-analysis of 60 randomized trials including 21,293 patients (CA-AKI incidence 10%) found forced matched diuresis (FMD) and hemodynamic-guided hydration superior strategies particularly in high-risk patients.[50] The more fluid administered (and therefore the more urine output increased), the greater the benefit. The timing of fluid administration is possibly confounded by how long it takes to increase urine output. Those studies supporting a prolonged preangiography fluid administration protocol used 0.9% saline alone, whereas the RenalGuard experience with supplemental IV furosemide suggests an hour or less preangiography is sufficient if urine output increases within that time frame.

A Unifying Hypothesis

The evidence suggests that the more fluid administered, the greater the benefit, and this is generally associated with an increase in urine output. The data from the PRINCE trial also found that the amount of urine output was inversely related to the incidence of CA-AKI.[32] How might an increase in urine output be the key to prevention of this form of AKI? The first explanation might be that increasing urine output decreases the concentration of a nephrotoxin within the tubule and also the contact time with tubule epithelium. While a satisfying explanation, there is little direct evidence to support this "dilution" hypothesis.

A second explanation is that increasing urine output in some way increases blood flow in the microvasculature of the kidney; this could occur in several ways. First the higher hydration volumes given to induce the high urine output may decrease the viscosity of the contrast media as it enters the small vessels of the kidney, in particular the vasa recti that supply blood to the oxygen-sensitive inner medulla of the kidney. In addition, there may be an indirect effect to increase vasa recti blood flow, mediated through intrarenal vasodilators. There is strong evidence in support of this as revealed in studies using blood oxygenation level–dependent MRI in humans,[51] urinary P_{O_2} measurements,[52] and direct oxygen-sensing probes in animals.[53] Drinking a lot of water acutely or administration of furosemide increases medullary oxygenation, an effect mediated in part by prostaglandin release within the kidney[51] and inhibition of oxygen consumption, respectively.[54] Using these same techniques, medullary oxygen level decreases during contrast administration in animals[55] and during TAVR[56] and CABG[57] and is predictive of subsequent AKI. Might increasing urine output particularly with furosemide during FMD mitigate that effect?

FINAL RECOMMENDATIONS

In all patients.

- Reduce NPO (nil per os) orders to 2 hours before procedure
- Encourage the consumption of water (at least 1 L) postprocedure
- Hold diuretics for at least 12 hours before procedure

In high-risk patients:

- Administer 0.9% NaCl
  - 250 mL immediately preprocedure (this is about 3 mL/kg)
  - 1 mL/kg/h during and after procedure (for 4–6 hours). This can be adjusted using LVEDP; CVP for higher rate

CONFLICTS OF INTEREST

R. Solomon is on the scientific advisory board for RenalGuard but has no financial interests in the company.

REFERENCES

1. Writing Committee M, Lawton JS, Tamis-Holland JE, et al. 2021 ACC/AHA/SCAI guideline for coronary artery revascularization: a report of the American College of Cardiology/American Heart Association Joint Committee on clinical

practice guidelines. J Am Coll Cardiol 2022;79(2):e21–129.

2. Kim et al. Am J Physiol Renal Physiol 286: F760-F766, 200.

3. Beran A, Altorok N, Srour O, et al. Balanced crystalloids versus normal saline in adults with sepsis: a comprehensive systematic review and meta-analysis. J Clin Med 2022;11(7).

4. Brown JR, McCullough PA, Splaine ME, et al. How do centres begin the process to prevent contrast-induced acute kidney injury: a report from a new regional collaborative. BMJ Qual Saf 2012;21(1):54–62.

5. Eisenberg RL, Bank WO, Hedgock MW. Renal failure after major angiography can be avoided with hydration. Am J Radiol 1981;136:859–61.

6. Chen S, Zhang J, Yei F, et al. Clinical outcomes of contrast-induced nephropathy in patients undergoing percutaneous coronary intervention: a prospective, multicenter, randomized study to analyze the effect of hydration and acetylcysteine. Int J Cardiol 2008;126:407–13.

7. Maioli M, Toso A, Leoncini M, et al. Sodium bicarbonate versus saline for the prevention of contrast-induced nephropathy in patients with renal dysfunction undergoing coronary angiography or intervention. J Am Coll Cardiol 2008;52(8):599–604.

8. Jurado-Roman A, Hernandez-Hernandez F, Garcia-Tejada J, et al. Role of hydration in contrast-induced nephropathy in patients who underwent primary percutaneous coronary intervention. Am J Cardiol 2015;115(9):1174–8.

9. Luo Y, Wang X, Ye Z, et al. Remedial hydration reduces the incidence of contrast-induced nephropathy and short-term adverse events in patients with ST-segment elevation myocardial infarction: a single-center, randomized trial. Intern Med 2014;53:2265–72.

10. Arslan S, Yildiz A, Dalgic Y, et al. Avoiding the emergence of contrast-induced acute kidney injury in acute coronary syndrome: routine hydration treatment. Coron Artery Dis 2021;32(5):397–402.

11. Jiang Y, Chen M, Zhang Y, et al. Meta-analysis of prophylactic hydration versus no hydration on contrast-induced acute kidney injury. Coron Artery Dis 2017;28(8):649–57.

12. Nijssen EC, Rennenberg RJ, Nelemans PJ, et al. Prophylactic hydration to protect renal function from intravascular iodinated contrast material in patients at high risk of contrast-induced nephropathy (AMACING): a prospective, randomized, phase 3, controlled, open-label, non-inferiority trial. Lancet 2017;389:1312–22.

13. Lee HC, Chuang KI, Lu CF, et al. Use of contrast Medium volume to Guide prophylactic hydration to prevent acute kidney injury after contrast administration: a meta-analysis. AJR Am J Roentgenol 2020;215(1):15–24.

14. Hiremath W, Akbari A, Shabana W, et al. Prevention of contrast-induced acute kidney injury: is simple oral hydration similar to intravenous? A systematic review of the evidence. PLoS One 2013;8:e60009.

15. Cheungpasitporn W, Thongprayoon C, Brabec BS, et al. Oral hydration for prevention of contrast-induced acute kidney injury in elective radiologic procedures: a systemic review and meta-analysis of randomized controlled trials. N Am J Med Sci 2014;6:618–24.

16. Agarwal SK, Mohareb S, Patel A, et al. Systematic oral hydration with water is similar to parenteral hydration for prevention of contrast-induced nephropathy: an updated meta-analysis of randomised clinical data. Open Heart 2015;2(1):e000317.

17. Zhang W, Zhang J, Yang B, et al. Effectiveness of oral hydration in preventing contrast-induced acute kidney injury in patients undergoing coronary angiography or intervention: a pairwise and network meta-analysis. Coron Artery Dis 2018;29(4):286–93.

18. Xie W, Zhou Y, Liao Z, et al. Effect of oral hydration on contrast-induced acute kidney injury among patients after primary percutaneous coronary intervention. Cardiorenal Med 2021;11(5–6):243–51.

19. Mueller C, Buerkle G, Buettner H, et al. Prevention of contrast media-associated nephropathy: randomized comparison of 2 hydration regimens in 1620 patients undergoing coronary angiography. Arch Int Med 2002;162:329–36.

20. Marron B, Ruiz E, Fernandez C, et al. Systemic and renal effects of preventing contrast nephrotoxicity with isotonic (0.9%) and hypotonic (045%) saline. Rev Esp Cardiol 2007;60:1018–25.

21. Merten G, Burgess WG, LV, et al. Prevention of contrast-induced nephropathy with sodium bicarbonate: a randomized controlled trial. JAMA 2004;291:2328–34.

22. Weisbord SD, Gallagher M, Jneid H, et al. Outcomes after angiography with sodium bicarbonate and acetylcysteine. N Engl J Med 2018;378(7):603–14.

23. Brar SS, Aharonian V, Mansukhani P, et al. Haemodynamic-guided fluid administration for the prevention of contrast-induced acute kidney injury: the POSEIDON randomised controlled trial. Lancet 2014;383(9931):1814–23.

24. Marashizadeh A, Sanati HR, Sadeghipour P, et al. Left ventricular end-diastolic pressure-guided hydration for the prevention of contrast-induced acute kidney injury in patients with stable ischemic heart disease: the LAKESIDE trial. Int Urol Nephrol 2019;51(10):1815–22.

25. Qian G, Fu Z, Guo J, et al. Prevention of contrast-induced nephropathy by central venous pressure-guided fluid administration in chronic kidney

disease and congestive heart failure patients. JACC Cardiovasc Interv 2016;9(1):89–96.

26. Maioli M, Toso A, Leoncini M, et al. Bioimpedance-guided hydration for the prevention of contrast-induced kidney injury: the HYDRA study. J Am Coll Cardiol 2018;71(25):2880–9.

27. Bei WJ, Wang K, Li HL, et al. Safe hydration to prevent contrast-induced acute kidney injury and worsening heart failure in patients with renal insufficiency and heart failure undergoing coronary angiography or percutaneous coronary intervention. Int Heart J 2019;60(2):247–54.

28. Soomro QH, Anand ST, Weisbord SD, et al. The relationship between rate and volume of intravenous fluid administration and kidney outcomes after angiography. Clin J Am Soc Nephrol 2022;17(10):1446–56.

29. Krasuski RA, Beard RM, Geoghagan JD, et al. Optimal timing of hydration to erase contrast-associated nephropathy: the other CAN study. J Invasive Cardiol 2003;15:699–702.

30. Taylor AJ, Hotchkiss D, Morse RW, et al. PREPARED: PREParation for angiography in REnal dysfunction. Chest 1998;114:1570–4.

31. Liu L, Zhou L, Li W, et al. Role of modified hydration for preventing contrast-associated acute kidney injury in patients with ST-segment elevation myocardial infarction after primary percutaneous coronary intervention. Intern Emerg Med 2022.

32. Stevens MA, McCullough P, Tobin K, et al. A prospective randomized trial of prevention measures in patients at high risk for contrast nephropathy. J Am Coll Cardiol 1999;33:403–11.

33. Briguori C, Visconti G, Donahue M, et al. RenalGuard system in high-risk patients for contrast-induced acute kidney injury. Am Heart J 2016;173:67–76.

34. Solomon R. Improving intravenous fluid therapy for prevention of contrast-induced nephropathy: how to give more without causing heart failure. JACC Cardiovasc Interv 2016;9(1):97–9.

35. Dussol B, Morange S, Loundoun A, et al. A randomized trial of saline hydration to prevent contrast nephropathy in chronic renal failure patients. Nephrol Dial Transplant 2006;21:2120–6.

36. Majumdar S, Kjellstrand CM, Tymchak WJ, et al. Forced euvolemic diuresis with mannitol and furosemide for prevention of contrast-induced nephropathy in patients with CKD undergoing coronary angiography: a randomized controlled trial. Am J Kid Dis 2009;54:602–9.

37. Solomon R, Werner C, Mann D, et al. Effects of saline, mannitol, and furosemide to prevent acute decreases in renal function induced by radiocontrast agents. N Engl J Med 1994;331:1416–20.

38. Weinstein JM, Heyman S, Brezis M. Potential deleterious effect of furosemide in radiocontrast nephropathy. Nephron 1992;62:413–5.

39. Gu GQ, Lu R, Cui W, et al. Low-dose furosemide administered with adequate hydration reduces contrast-induced nephropathy in patients undergoing coronary angiography. Cardiology 2013;125(2):69–73.

40. Hu M, Yan G, Tang H, et al. Effect of combining furosemide with standard hydration therapy on contrast-induced acute kidney injury following coronary angiography or intervention in a high-risk population. Angiology 2021;72(2):138–44.

41. Barbanti M, Gulino S, Capranzano P, et al. Acute kidney injury with the RenalGuard system in patients undergoing transcatheter aortic valve Replacement: the PROTECT-TAVI trial (PROphylactic effecT of furosEmide-induCed diuresis with matched isotonic intravenous hydraTion in transcatheter aortic valve implantation). JACC Cardiovasc Interv 2015;8(12):1595–604.

42. Bertelli L, Politi L, Roversi S, et al. Comparison of RenalGuard system, continuous venovenous hemofiltration and hydration inhigh-risk patients for contrast-induced nephropathy. JACC (J Am Coll Cardiol) 2012;59:E96.

43. Briguori C. Renalguard system: a dedicated device to prevent contrast-induced acute kidney injury. Int J Cardiol 2013;168(2):643–4.

44. Briguori C, Visconti G, Focaccio A, et al. Renal insufficiency after contrast media administration trial II (REMEDIAL II): RenalGuard system in high-risk patients for contrast-induced acute kidney injury. Circulation 2011;124(11):1260–9.

45. Resnic F, Davidson CJ, Zelman R, et al. Prevention of contrast induced nephropathy using high volume matched diuresis using the RenalGuard system: first-in-man study. J Am Coll Cardiol 2009;53:A36.

46. Visconti G, Focaccio A, Donahue M, et al. RenalGuard system for the prevention of acute kidney injury in patients undergoing transcatheter aortic valve implantation. EuroIntervention 2016;11(14):e1658–61.

47. Wang Y, Guo Y. RenalGuard system and conventional hydration for preventing contrast-associated acute kidney injury in patients undergoing cardiac interventional procedures: a systematic review and meta-analysis. Int J Cardiol 2021;333:83–9.

48. Briguori C, D'Amore C, De Micco F, et al. Left ventricular end-diastolic pressure versus urine flow rate-guided hydration in preventing contrast-associated acute kidney injury. JACC Cardiovasc Interv 2020;13(17):2065–74.

49. Mirza AJ, Ali K, Huwez F, et al. Contrast induced nephropathy: efficacy of matched hydration and forced diuresis for prevention in patients with impaired renal function undergoing coronary procedures-CINEMA trial. Int J Cardiol Heart Vasc 2022;39:100959.

50. Cai Q, Jing R, Zhang W, et al. Hydration strategies for preventing contrast-induced acute kidney injury: a systematic review and Bayesian network meta-analysis. J Interv Cardiol 2020;2020:7292675.

51. Prasad PV, Epstein FH. Changes in renal medullary pO2 during water diuresis as evaluated by blood oxygenation level-dependent magnetic resonance imaging: effects of aging and cyclooxygenase inhibition. Kidney Int 1999;55(1):294–8.

52. Evans RG, Smith JA, Wright C, et al. Urinary oxygen tension: a clinical window on the health of the renal medulla? Am J Physiol Regul Integr Comp Physiol 2014;306(1):R45–50.

53. Prasad P, Edelman RR, Epstein FH. Noninvasive evaluation of intrarenal oxygenation with BOLD MRI. Circulation 1996;94:3271–8.

54. Epstein FH, Prasad P. Effects of furosemide on medullary oxygenation in younger and older subjects. Kidney Int 2000;57(5):2080–3.

55. Li LP, Franklin T, Du H, et al. Intrarenal oxygenation by blood oxygenation level-dependent MRI in contrast nephropathy model: effect of the viscosity and dose. J Magn Reson Imaging 2012;36(5):1162–7.

56. Dae MW, Liu KD, Solomon RJ, et al. Effect of low-frequency therapeutic ultrasound on induction of nitric oxide in CKD: potential to prevent acute kidney injury. Kidney Dis 2020;1–8.

57. Zhu MZL, Martin A, Cochrane AD, et al. Urinary hypoxia: an intraoperative marker of risk of cardiac surgery-associated acute kidney injury. Nephrol Dial Transplant 2018.

A Practical Approach to Preventing Contrast-Associated Renal Complications in the Catheterization Laboratory

Hitinder S. Gurm, MBBS*

KEYWORDS

- Contrast-induced acute kidney injury • Ultra-low contrast volume
- Renal function-based contrast dosing

KEY POINTS

- Contrast-associated acute kidney injury (CA-AKI) is a key concern among patients undergoing coronary angiography and percutaneous coronary interventions.
- The key steps for the prevention of CA-AKI remain avoiding dehydration, adequate hydration, and contrast minimization.
- In patients with Stage IV chronic kidney disease, ultra-low contrast procedure (contrast dose $\leq$ GFR) may be especially beneficial.

Contrast media are administered daily in every catheterization laboratory around the world, and it is impossible to fathom contemporary diagnostic or interventional practice without the availability of iodinated contrast media. Indeed, the central role of contrast media in contemporary practice (if there was ever any doubt) became clear secondary to disruptions in care that resulted from supply change disruptions and nationwide shortage of certain contrast media during the COVID pandemic.

While contrast media are generally safe, they are like any other drug and do carry some risk. Two categories of risk are important to consider when using contrast media in the catheterization laboratory; renal toxicity and immune-mediated reactions. Every team member working in the catheterization laboratory needs to be aware of these risks and every facility should have clear protocols to prevent or respond to these complications.

Practically, a catheterization laboratory needs to have clear protocols to ensure renal safety and established protocols and readiness to manage allergic reactions. The goal of this article is to discuss a practical approach for preventing contrast-associated renal complications. Severe allergic reactions are rare in the catheterization laboratory but can be fatal if not addressed in a timely manner. The reader is advised to consider the excellent resources available elsewhere for developing a state of readiness for responding to such a reaction (see BMC2 best practice protocols available at: https://bmc2.org/quality-improvement/best-practices).

Contrast-associated acute kidney injury (CA-AKI) is a well-recognized complication among patients undergoing coronary angiography or

Conflict of Interest: H.S. Gurm receives research support from Blue Cross Blue Shield of Michigan. He is the co-founder of, owns equity in, and is a consultant to Amplitude Vascular Systems. He also owns equity in Jiaxing Bossh Medical Technology Partnership and has previously consulted for Osprey Medical. He is the chair of the Clinical Events Committee for the PERFORMANCE trial sponsored by Contego Medical.
Internal Medicine, University of Michigan, Ann Arbor, MI, USA
* Frankel Cardiovascular Center, 2A 192F, 1500 East Medical Ctr Drive, Ann Arbor, MI 48109-5853.
E-mail address: hgurm@med.umich.edu

Percutaneous Coronary Intervention (PCI) and is associated with increased mortality, morbidity, and health care expense.[1,2] While there was a broader consensus on the importance of renal toxicity of contrast media in the first few decades of interventional practice, more recently, perspectives have started to diverge on the relevance of CA-AKI in contemporary practice. On one extreme is the argument that contrast media have no renal toxicity,[3] and at the other extreme, there is evidence of "renalism," where patients with abnormal renal functions are denied indicated diagnostic or therapeutic procedures with a resultant increase in morbidity and potentially mortality.[4] A careful analysis of the data would suggest that neither of the views is entirely correct: contrast-induced kidney injury is a real entity, but the true risk of contrast-induced kidney injury has been overestimated in the recent literature. Healthy animals exposed to contrast in large doses develop AKI in a predictable fashion, thus supporting an association between high contrast dose and renal toxicity.[5] There is indirect evidence to suggest that human kidneys behave similarly and in observational studies, patients exposed to higher doses of contrast media are more likely to develop AKI. Conversely, patients with chronic kidney disease who undergo zero contrast or ultra-low contrast PCI have a much lower likelihood of developing AKI than those receiving higher doses of contrast, supporting a robust association between contrast media dose and the risk of AKI.[6,7] Finally, community efforts to reduce contrast media dosing have translated into reduction in rates of AKI suggesting that a low contrast dose is safe and desirable goal.[8]

The three key steps, endorsed by professional society guidelines for the prevention of CA-AKI are based on fundamental toxicology principles and constitute identifying patients at the highest risk, ensuring adequate hydration and contrast minimization. Tubular toxicity from contrast media is nonlinearly associated with the amount of contrast delivered to the renal tubule and patients with low GFR whether chronic as seen in chronic kidney disease or acute, as seen with hypovolemia or shock are more prone to renal injury from contrast. The same principle likely explains the association between renal function-based contrast dose and renal toxicity of contrast media.

The risk factors for CI-AKI are well recognized, and numerous groups, including ours, have developed risk models with varying degrees of accuracy and sophistication.[9] One common feature of these models is that they have found little to limited clinical applicability. The

most likely reason for this may be that most decisions in the catheterization laboratory follow the *fast-and-frugal heuristics framework* and information that forces a binary decision is more likely to be adopted into practice, than more complex risk models.[10] In addition, no large study has successfully demonstrated the ability of risk-based approach to care to translate into clinically meaningful change in outcomes.

We recommend one of the 2 approaches for risk stratification. The simplest and easiest to implement as part of a regular workflow is to ensure visibility of the estimated glomerular filtration rate (eGFR) before the procedure. This can be done at the procedure time out and ensures that the entire team is aware of the patients risk and the predicted contrast thresholds. The second is to embed an automated risk calculator in the EMR. Some organizations have successfully done that and include such risk stratification as part of the procedural consent and in identifying patients who might be candidates for ultra-low contrast dosing. It is important to recognize that the majority of models for CA-AKI have poor discrimination and if an organization elects to embed a risk prediction model in their workflow, they should specifically use a model with a high level of discrimination. Some of the best models are available free from the investigators who developed them. We have previously endorsed the BMC2/SCAI risk model[11] but this model is nearly a decade old and in the absence of published data on its calibration in contemporary practice, it is not possible to recommend this model versus any of the more recent models.[12]

The second key principle to consider is hydration. For nearly 3 decades, hydration has been the cornerstone of CA-AKI prevention, but this hypothesis has been tested in recent studies. Despite early excitement that followed the initial work, clinical investigations of intravenous (IV) sodium bicarbonate, hypothesized to ameliorate oxidative stress via urine alkalinization, showed no benefit versus saline.[13,14] Subsequent studies targeted IV volume expansion, with favorable results for hemodynamic guided and diuretic matched hydration strategies.[15,16] Given the simplicity and the strong data, left ventricular end diastolic pressure (LVEDP) guided hydration has become the standard in many laboratories. In parallel, however, challenges to the IV volume expansion hypothesis have also arisen, with multiple studies demonstrating the safety of no-hydration, minimal IV hydration, or oral hydration only, strategies in select populations.[17,18] In the absence of clear data favoring any one strategy, the 2018 ESC and 2021 ACC/AHA/SCAI revascularization guidelines advocate for adequate hydration and allow for tailored strategies to reduce risk of CA-AKI.[19–23]

Based on this emerging data, we believe that most patients can forego pre-hydration as long as dehydration is avoided. This can be achieved safely by foregoing pre-procedure nil per os (NPO) order and encouraging patients to drink clear water up to 2 hours prior to the procedure. We follow oral pre-hydration by LVEDP-based hydration for postprocedure hydration.

The final approach to renal safety is contrast minimization. Two different approaches to contrast dosing have been advocated, a renal function-based contrast dosing where an attempt is made to complete the procedure with contrast volume less than thrice the creatinine clearance or a risk model-based contrast

dosing.[24] We prefer the simpler renal function-based contrast threshold due to its simplicity and widespread and ready applicability. Many of the leading catheterization laboratories include GFR and the contrast thresholds of 1 X eGFR, 2 X eGFR, and 3 X eGFR and that simple step has been effective at lowering the total contrast volume that is routinely administered. While device-based approaches have been successful at minimizing the total contrast administered to the patient, the cost-effectiveness of such an approach remains to be established.[25]

The benefit of ultra-low contrast (<1 X eGFR) is most evident in the highest risk patients[6] and we reserve the use of ultra-low contrast for patients with CKD Stage 4. Some operators have perfected the art of no contrast PCI but it remains available only at select centers. At the moment the risk-benefit of ultra-low versus no contrast procedures remains unclear.

Conclusion: Despite a large number of studies evaluating devices and drug therapies, the key steps for the prevention of CA-AKI remain avoiding dehydration, adequate hydration, and contrast minimization. Box 1 provides a simplified approach to the prevention of CA-AKI in the catheterization laboratory.

CLINICS CARE POINTS

- Implementation of preventive strategies is key to reducing contrast-induced acute kidney injury.

- eGFR acknowledgment in the time out is a useful practice that grounds the entire team on procedure risk.

- Avoiding Dehydration is key, Adopt a hydration protocol using a combination of oral and intravenous hydration, especially for the highest risk patients.

- Limit contrast volume to less than 2 to 3 times the eGFR for all patients, and attempt to use ultra-low contrast volume in highest-risk patients

---

Box 1
A simplified protocol for the prevention of Contrast-Associated Acute kidney injury

Pre -procedure

1. Avoid NPO for longer than 2 hours for liquids. Encourage patient to drink 1 glass of water between 2 and 3 hours prior to the procedure.

2. Stop NSAIDs at least 24 hours prior to the procedure.

During the Procedure

1. Confirm GFR during the procedure time out.

2. Confirm eGFR- and eGFR-based contrast volume thresholds (2 X and 3 X eGFR) in the procedure time out; aim for contrast volume $<$ 2 to 3 X eGFR

3. In high-risk patients, (eGFR $<$ 30 ml/min/1.73m^2), or predicted risk of AKI $>$ 7%), consider ultra-low- contrast volume procedure if feasible (contrast volume $<$ 1 X eGFR); use IVUS guidance instead of contrast guidance

Post Procedure

1. Hydrate based on the LVEDP as per the POSEDION protocol.

LVEDP less than 13 mm Hg- 5 mL/kg/h x 4 hours

LVEDP 13 mm Hg to 18 mm Hg - 3 mL/kg/h for 4 hours

LVEDP greater than 18 mm Hg - 1.5 mL/kg/h for 4 hours

For patients weighing greater than 100kg, use a body weight of 100kg for the calculation of hydration volume

---

REFERENCES

1. Tsai TT, Patel UD, Chang TI, et al. Contemporary incidence, predictors, and outcomes of acute kidney injury in patients undergoing percutaneous coronary interventions: insights from the NCDR Cath-PCI registry. JACC Cardiovasc Interv 2014;7: 1–9.

2. Kooiman J, Seth M, Nallamothu BK, et al. Association between acute kidney injury and in-hospital mortality in patients undergoing percutaneous coronary interventions. Circ Cardiovasc Interv 2015;8: e002212.

3. Ehrmann S, Aronson D, Hinson JS. Contrast-associated acute kidney injury is a myth: Yes. Intensive Care Med 2018;44:104–6.

4. Chertow GM, Normand SL, McNeil BJ. "Renalism": inappropriately low rates of coronary angiography in elderly individuals with renal insufficiency. J Am Soc Nephrol 2004;15:2462–8.

5. Lauver DA, Carey EG, Bergin IL, et al. Sildenafil citrate for prophylaxis of nephropathy in an animal model of contrast-induced acute kidney injury. PLoS One 2014;9:e113598.

6. Gurm HS, Seth M, Dixon SR, et al. Contemporary use of and outcomes associated with ultra-low contrast volume in patients undergoing percutaneous coronary interventions. Catheter Cardiovasc Interv 2019;93:222–30.

7. Almendarez M, Gurm HS, Mariani J Jr, et al. Procedural Strategies to Reduce the Incidence of Contrast-Induced Acute Kidney Injury During Percutaneous Coronary Intervention. JACC Cardiovasc Interv 2019;12:1877–88.

8. Gurm HS, Seth M, Dixon S, et al. Trends in Contrast Volume Use and Incidence of Acute Kidney Injury in Patients Undergoing Percutaneous Coronary Intervention: Insights From Blue Cross Blue Shield of Michigan Cardiovascular Collaborative (BMC2). JACC Cardiovasc Interv 2018;11: 509–11.

9. Kooiman J, Gurm HS. Predicting Contrast-induced Renal Complications in the Catheterization Laboratory. Interventional cardiology clinics 2014;3: 369–77.

10. Marewski JN, Gigerenzer G. Heuristic decision making in medicine. Dialogues Clin Neurosci 2012;14:77.

11. Gurm HS, Seth M, Kooiman J, et al. A novel tool for reliable and accurate prediction of renal complications in patients undergoing percutaneous coronary intervention. J Am Coll Cardiol 2013;61: 2242–8.

12. Mehran R, Owen R, Chiarito M, et al. A contemporary simple risk score for prediction of contrast-associated acute kidney injury after percutaneous coronary intervention: derivation and validation from an observational registry. Lancet 2021;398:1974–83.

13. Merten GJ, Burgess WP, Gray LV, et al. Prevention of contrast-induced nephropathy with sodium bicarbonate: a randomized controlled trial. JAMA 2004;291:2328–34.

14. Brar SS, Shen AY, Jorgensen MB, et al. Sodium bicarbonate vs sodium chloride for the prevention of contrast medium-induced nephropathy in patients undergoing coronary angiography: a randomized trial. JAMA 2008;300:1038–46.

15. Brar SS, Aharonian V, Mansukhani P, et al. Haemodynamic-guided fluid administration for the prevention of contrast-induced acute kidney injury: the POSEIDON randomised controlled trial. Lancet 2014;383:1814–23.

16. Moroni F, Baldetti L, Kabali C, et al. Tailored Versus Standard Hydration to Prevent Acute Kidney Injury After Percutaneous Coronary Intervention: Network Meta-Analysis. J Am Heart Assoc 2021;10:e021342.

17. Timal RJ, Kooiman J, Sijpkens YWJ, et al. Effect of No Prehydration vs Sodium Bicarbonate Prehydration Prior to Contrast-Enhanced Computed Tomography in the Prevention of Postcontrast Acute Kidney Injury in Adults With Chronic Kidney Disease: The Kompas Randomized Clinical Trial. JAMA Intern Med 2020;180: 533–41.

18. Nijssen EC, Rennenberg RJ, Nelemans PJ, et al. Prophylactic hydration to protect renal function from intravascular iodinated contrast material in patients at high risk of contrast-induced nephropathy (AMACING): a prospective, randomised, phase 3, controlled, open-label, non-inferiority trial. Lancet 2017;389:1312–22.

19. Sousa-Uva M, Neumann FJ, Ahlsson A, et al. 2018 ESC/EACTS Guidelines on myocardial revascularization. Eur J Cardio Thorac Surg 2019;55:4–90.

20. Writing Committee M, Lawton JS, Tamis-Holland JE, et al. 2021 ACC/AHA/SCAI Guideline for Coronary Artery Revascularization: Executive Summary: A Report of the American College of Cardiology/American Heart Association Joint Committee on Clinical Practice Guidelines. J Am Coll Cardiol 2022;79:197–215.

21. Writing Committee M, Lawton JS, Tamis-Holland JE, et al. 2021 ACC/AHA/SCAI Guideline for Coronary Artery Revascularization: A Report of the American College of Cardiology/American Heart Association Joint Committee on Clinical Practice Guidelines. J Am Coll Cardiol 2022;79: e21–129.

22. Lawton JS, Tamis-Holland JE, Bangalore S, et al. 2021 ACC/AHA/SCAI Guideline for Coronary Artery Revascularization: Executive Summary: A Report of the American College of Cardiology/American Heart Association Joint Committee on Clinical Practice Guidelines. Circulation 2022;145: e4–17.

23. Lawton JS, Tamis-Holland JE, Bangalore S, et al. 2021 ACC/AHA/SCAI Guideline for Coronary Artery Revascularization: A Report of the American College of Cardiology/American Heart Association

Joint Committee on Clinical Practice Guidelines. Circulation 2022;145:e18–114.

24. Gurm HS, Dixon SR, Smith DE, et al. Renal function-based contrast dosing to define safe limits of radiographic contrast media in patients undergoing percutaneous coronary interventions. J Am Coll Cardiol 2011;58:907–14.

25. Gurm HS, Mavromatis K, Bertolet B, et al. Minimizing radiographic contrast administration during coronary angiography using a novel contrast reduction system: A multicenter observational study of the DyeVert plus contrast reduction system. Catheter Cardiovasc Interv 2019;93:1228–35.

Implications of Kidney Disease in Patients with Peripheral Arterial Disease and Vascular Calcification

Yogamaya Mantha, MD, Anum Asif, MD,
Ayman Fath, MD, Anand Prasad, MD, FSCAI, RPVI*

KEYWORDS

- Chronic kidney disease • Medial calcification • Critical limb ischemia • Peripheral arterial disease
- Peripheral vascular intervention • Atherectomy • Intravascular lithotripsy

KEY POINTS

- PAD is described to occur due to atherosclerotic plaques causing blockage.
- Calcification occurs frequently concomitant with the progression of these atherosclerotic plaques in the intimal layer.
- Patients with chronic kidney disease (CKD) have a higher risk of developing atherosclerosis and PAD than age-matched individuals with normal kidney function.
- Among patients with CKD, calcification of the medial layer of arterial vessels is the major form of vascular calcification (VC) and cause of PAD in addition to intimal atherosclerosis and calcification.
- Traditional cardiovascular (CV) risk factors such as diabetes mellitus (DM), hypertension, and tobacco use, patients with CKD have nontraditional CV risk factors such as uremia, inflammation, and disorders of mineral metabolism that play an important role in the pathogenesis of PAD.

INTRODUCTION

Peripheral arterial disease (PAD) is a progressive occlusive disorder of peripheral arteries supplying arms, legs as well as aorta. Classically, PAD is described to occur due to atherosclerotic plaques causing blockage.[1,2] However, calcification occurs frequently concomitant with the progression of these atherosclerotic plaques in the intimal layer. Patients with chronic kidney disease (CKD) have a higher risk of developing atherosclerosis and PAD than age-matched individuals with normal kidney function.[3,4] Among patients with CKD, calcification of the medial layer of arterial vessels is the major form of vascular calcification (VC) and cause of PAD in addition to intimal atherosclerosis and calcification. In addition to traditional cardiovascular (CV) risk factors such as diabetes mellitus (DM), hypertension, and tobacco use, patients with CKD have nontraditional CV risk factors such as uremia, inflammation, and disorders of mineral metabolism that play an important role in the pathogenesis of PAD.[4,5] The present review provides an overview of PAD, specifically the pathophysiology and clinical challenges posed by extensive VC present in patients with CKD.

Division of Cardiology, Department of Medicine, UT Health San Antonio, MC 7872, 8300 Floyd Curl Drive, San Antonio, TX 78229-3900, USA
* Corresponding author. Division of Cardiology, Department of Medicine, Vascular Medicine, UT Health San Antonio.
E-mail address: prasada@uthscsa.edu
Twitter: @AnandPrasadMD (A.P.)

Intervent Cardiol Clin 12 (2023) 531–538
https://doi.org/10.1016/j.iccl.2023.06.010
2211-7458/23/© 2023 Elsevier Inc. All rights reserved.

EPIDEMIOLOGY OF PERIPHERAL ARTERY DISEASE IN CHRONIC KIDNEY DISEASE

The US National Health and Nutrition Examination Survey have reported the prevalence of PAD in patients with DM to be 3-fold higher than those without DM, whereas the risk of PAD increased by 6.5 times in patients with estimated glomerular filtration rate (eGFR) < 60 mL/min/1.73 m^2 as compared with eGFR ≥60 mL/min/1.73 m^2.[6] In a large meta-analysis of more than 800,000 patients in the CKD-Prognosis Consortium, the risk for developing PAD increased by 22% for eGFR of 45 mL/min/1.73 m^2 and by 2-fold for eGFR of 15 mL/min/1.73 m^2 compared to eGFR of 90 mL/min/1.73 m^2. Similarly, the risk increased by 50% for albuminuria of 30 mg/g and by about 2-fold for albuminuria of 300 mg/g compared to albuminuria of 5 mg/g.[7] Moreover, nearly half of patients with ESRD starting dialysis have subclinical or overt PAD.[2,3]

PATHOPHYSIOLOGY OF PERIPHERAL ARTERY DISEASE AND VASCULAR CALCIFICATION IN CHRONIC KIDNEY DISEASE

The cause–effect relationship between kidney function and PAD risk has been extensively studied. The traditional risk factors such as DM, hypertension, obesity, and smoking are highly prevalent in CKD population and contribute to PAD risk. Moreover, renal impairment independently contributes to increased risk via multiple mechanisms including increased production of proinflammatory cytokines, oxidative stress, endothelial dysfunction, volume expansion, and the uremic toxins.[8] In addition, altered bone-mineral metabolism in advanced CKD with high-phosphorous and -calcium milieu causing abnormalities of parathyroid hormone (PTH), and fibroblast growth factor-23 (FGF23) are the other important players. Perticone and colleagues[9] found a significant inverse relationship between alkaline phosphatase and endothelium-dependent vasodilation, mediated by an increase in FGF23 which is an early marker of endothelial dysfunction in patients with CKD. Albuminuria is considered a biomarker of endothelial injury and dysfunction.[1,10] In the retrospective cohort, albuminuria has been associated with increased pulse pressure, high transcapillary escape rate of fibrinogen, and elevated levels of von Willebrand factor. All these factors represent endothelial dysfunction and can lead to impairment of kidney over time amplifying pro-inflammatory and pro-fibrotic pathways.[11] Moreover, the excess albumin filtered through the glomerular capillaries has a direct toxic effect on renal tubules exacerbating the tubular and glomerular damage. Thus, it is demonstrated that CKD and albuminuria are independent risk factors for atherosclerosis and PAD. The pathophysiology of cardiovascular and kidney disease relationship has been extensively discussed in Mehta and colleagues' article, "Significance of Kidney Disease in Cardiovascular Disease Patients," in this issue.

In populations with traditional risk factors but normal renal function, VC is a chronic advance atherosclerotic plaque accumulation that occurs within the intimal layer. Atheromatous intimal calcification occurs due to cellular necrosis, inflammation, and lipid deposition. It exhibits a more sporadic and discontinuous course along the artery and is often associated with negative remodeling. Mechanisms that contribute to intimal calcification, such as shear stress, local inflammation, oxidative stress to the endothelium, and the calcification of macrophage and vascular smooth muscle cell-derived microvesicles, are amplified in patients with CKD.[12,13] Moreover, in CKD, the calcification of the medial layer of the artery is a distinct added phenomenon and is associated with the duration of kidney disease, calcium–phosphate disorders, albuminuria, diabetes, and ageing (Fig. 1). Medial calcification occurs along the internal elastic lamina and causes loss of vessel elasticity, resulting in increased systolic blood pressure, lower diastolic pressures and left ventricle hypertrophy which may ultimately lead to increased CV morbidity and mortality. In patients undergoing chronic hemodialysis, intimal and medial calcification develops rapidly.[14]

Medical calcification is a complex intracellular molecular process involving the differentiation of macrophages and vascular smooth muscle cells (VSMCs) into non-collagen proteins producing cells such as osteoclast-like cells, similar to biomineralization in bone formation.[14,15] Moreover, medications used to control phosphate homeostasis, often used in patients with CKD to treat hyperphosphatemia and secondary hyperparathyroidism, have been reported to have an inverse relationship to the extent of vessel calcification.[16,17] Several studies demonstrated that the administration of calcium-containing phosphate binders used with vitamin D analogs, often goes along with an excess calcium load and is found to be associated with the progression of VC.[18,19] In addition, several inhibitors of the calcification process are dysregulated in this cohort. Matrix

Medial Calcification (Concentric)
- Disordered mineral metabolism
- Increased calcium phosphate particles
- Increased oxidative stress
- Inflammatory cytokines
- Medial fibrosis and elastinolysis

Atherosclerotic Intimal Calcification (Eccentric)
- Subintimal lipid deposition
- Lipid oxidation
- Inflammatory cytokines

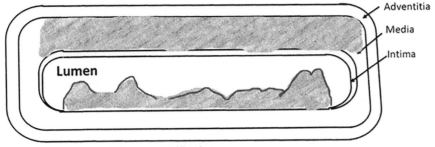

Causes of Vascular Calcification
- CKD, Dialysis, Diabetes
- Disorders of bone mineralization such as hyperphosphatemia
- Hormonal disorders
- Medications: Vitamin D, Senelamer, Denosumab
- Loss of inhibitors: Matrix Gla protein, fetuin-A, and pyrophosphate

Fig. 1. Schematic diagram depicting multiple mechanisms leading to vascular calcification.

Gla protein, fetuin-A, and pyrophosphate mainly prevent the formation of calcium phosphate crystals in vessels. In dialysis patients, circulating fetuin-A32 and pyrophosphate are reduced compared to healthy subjects.[20,21]

A third and rare form of VC is calcific uremic arteriolopathy (CUA) or calciphylaxis, which is characterized by diffuse peripheral calcification including soft tissues.[22] CUA most often occurs in adult dialysis patients with diabetes, obesity, hyperphosphatemia, on medications such as warfarin, calcium-based phosphate binders, and long dialysis vintage. Calcification, in particular AIC and severely calcified lesions, pose challenges for both surgical and endovascular therapy and have an increased risk for restenosis.

CRITICAL LIMB ISCHEMIA

The American Heart Association (AHA)/American College of Cardiology (ACC) guidelines for lower-extremity PAD define critical limb ischemia (CLI) as the presence of ischemic rest pain, nonhealing wound/ulcer, or gangrene for >2 weeks with associated evidence of hypoperfusion as measured by ankle-brachial index (ABI), toe-brachial index (TBI), transcutaneous oximetry, or skin perfusion pressure.[23] CLI is considered the most severe form of PAD and is often seen in patients with CKD and DM. Evidence has shown that patients with CLI have

higher mortality rates than patients with symptomatic coronary artery disease.[24] Thus, prompt diagnosis and treatment with revascularization is a Class I indication in the AHA/ACC guidelines in order to reduce major and minor amputations and other subsequent complications.[2]

DIAGNOSTIC IMAGING OF PERIPHERAL ARTERY DISEASE AND CRITICAL LIMB ISCHEMIA IN PATIENTS WITH CHRONIC KIDNEY DISEASE

Several noninvasive imaging techniques, including computed tomographic (CT) and magnetic resonance (MR) imaging, duplex ultrasonography, measurement of pulse wave velocity, planar radiographs, ABI and TBI are available for the detection of peripheral calcification and PAD. However, PAD is still underrecognized and under diagnosed. According to the PART-NERS study (Peripheral Arterial Disease Awareness, Risk, and Treatment: New Resources for Survival) including elderly or patients 50-70 years age with either history of smoking or diabetes, 83% of patients had a prior PAD diagnosis, yet only 49% of their physicians were aware of it.[25] ABI is considered first line to detect PAD and a score of 0.9 has sensitivity and specificity, of 61% to 73% and 83% to 96%, respectively.[26] However, ABIs may be limited due to medial artery calcification in patients with CKD that causes decreased arterial compliance, elevated pressures and thus falsely elevated values. In this context, toe-brachial index (TBI) can be used as medial calcification rarely affects digital arteries.[2,27] A TBI ≤0.70 is accepted as the diagnostic value for PAD.[2] In a review of prospectively collected data, the sensitivity and overall accuracy for detecting 50% of greater stenosis were evaluated for ABI and TBI in patients with CKD versus non-CKD. For ABI, the corresponding values were 60% (95% CI, 56.3–64.6) and 76% (95% CI, 73.1–78.1) in patients without CKD versus 43% (95% CI, 34.3–52.7) and 67% (95% CI, 60.2–73.0) in CKD. On contrary, these values for TBI were 77% (95% CI, 61.4–88.2) and 72% (95% CI, 59.9–82.3) for patients with CKD.[28] In a recent analysis, the difference between ABI and TBI was evaluated to capture both PAD and medial calcification. In patients with CKD with ABI values ≥ 0.9, ABI-TBI values greater than the median were associated with greater risk for all-cause mortality.[29] Thus, the simultaneous measurement of ABI and TBI in patients with diabetes or CKD might prove useful.

Exercise treadmill ABI testing is useful in establishing the diagnosis of lower extremity PAD in symptomatic patients with normal resting (1–1.4) or borderline (0.91–0.99) ABI values, but can be limited in patients with foot ulcers or gangrene. CT and MR with angiography are highly sensitive methods to assess the anatomy, degree, and extent of VC and arterial stenosis. However, both imaging modalities use contrast agents (iodinated for computed tomography and gadolinium-based for MR), which are associated with nephrotoxicity and nephrogenic systemic fibrosis (NSF), respectively. Moreover, CTA is limited in the diagnosis of PAD in small tibial vessels with calcification and multiple occlusions. The recent development of 256-row CTA has made detecting stenosis in the tibial location possible however with the exemption of patients with severe calcific disease.[30] MRA has several advantages over CTA in diagnosing PAD. For example, MRA does not require radiation, calcification does not interfere with the imaging technique, and it can be used to perform hemodynamic assessments.[23] As mentioned earlier there has been a concern of gadolinium-induced NSF in patients with ESRD; however, the latest ACR-NKF (American College of Radiology–National Kidney Foundation) consensus report states that risk of NSF from group 2 gadolinium agents is very low and a procedure should not be held or delayed if harm would result from not proceeding with an indicated contrast-enhanced MRI.[31]

Catheter-based angiography remains the gold standard diagnostic test for PAD as it can assess the anatomy, perform hemodynamic assessments and provide an opportunity for intervention. New techniques are available that help to reduce the use of iodinated contrast. CTA and MRA imaging may be incorporated to the angiogram, which may have the potential to reduce the use of contrast and radiation. Alternatively, CO_2 angiography is hypothesized as a replacement or supplement to reduce contrast of conventional contrast-based angiography. However, according to Ghumman et all, CO_2-based angiography was still associated with high incidence of acute kidney injury at 6.2% and other nonrenal adverse side effects.[32]

PERIPHERAL VASCULAR INTERVENTION IN PATIENTS WITH CHRONIC KIDNEY DISEASE

Currently, there is no specific proven pharmacotherapy to prevent progression or facilitate regression of VC. Preliminary experimental data on magnesium, vitamin K, and sodium thiosulfate therapies were successful; however, failed to demonstrate improvement in VC in clinical trials.[34–36] In the presence of severe calcific plaque, revascularization is challenging and is known to portend lower success rates, increased complications, and the rates of re-stenosis, which decreases overall clinical outcomes.[33] In addition, vessel recoil, dissection, distal embolization, and perforation are potential complications that affect short- and long-term clinical outcomes. Current advances in endovascular technology continue to expand the patient subsets that can be treated with peripheral endovascular intervention (PVI). In a large observational study, PVI compared with surgery was associated with reduced in-hospital mortality (2.34% versus 2.73%, P < 0.001), length of stay (8.7 days versus 10.7 days, P < 0.001), and cost of hospitalization ($31,679 versus $32,485, P < 0.001) despite similar rates of major amputation (6.5% versus 5.7%, P = 0.75).[37] According to Garimella and colleagues in a large review on the in-hospital outcomes of post-revascularization in hemodialysis patients, there were 77,049 PVI and 29,556 surgical procedures in which post-procedure complication rates nearly doubled in those undergoing surgery. In addition, there was an overall decrease in surgical procedures and an increase in PVI.[38] More recently data from the BEST-CLI study demonstrated that in selected patients with CLI with usable native saphenous veins, bypass surgery may

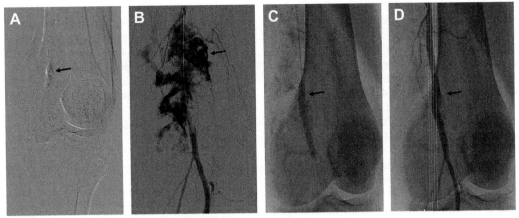

Fig. 2. (A), Lower extremity angiogram showing large, near occlusive, calcific plaque in the mid portion of the left popliteal artery; (B), Directional atherectomy was performed complicated by left popliteal artery perforation. (C and D), After 10 minutes of balloon tamponade, a 6 mm × 2.5 cm self-expanding covered stent was successfully deployed.

be superior to endovascular therapy at limb salvage. In this study, the cohort who did not have suitable vein (synthetic conduit), had no differences between endovascular or surgical therapy. In this both cohorts, the presence of renal dysfunction or dialysis dependence did not favor one therapy over the other.[39]

VC poses a significant mechanical concern for vessel treatment during PVI procedures. Atherectomy is a PVI technique that uses directional, orbital or rotational, excisional or aspiration, or laser technologies to debulk stenotic and occlusive calcific lesions.[40] The debulking process may allow for a more uniform angioplasty result with minimal vessel barotrauma and improved luminal diameter, thereby decreasing complications and vessel remodeling.[41] Furthermore, the presence

of VC may limit the delivery of drug-coated balloon therapies. While atherectomy has shown to improve device delivery, few randomized data are available to support routine use.

Data comparing atherectomy with other endovascular treatments for PAD, in patients with CKD, have shown similar patency rates with lower bailout stenting.[42–44] However, the risk for distal embolization is significantly higher with atherectomy when compared to only balloon angioplasty.[43] Intravascular lithotripsy (IVL) is a novel therapy for the treatment of VC. IVL technology (Shockwave Medical, Santa Clara, CA) is currently available for clinical use in the coronary and peripheral vascular beds. IVL technology with the incorporation of lithotripsy emitters on the shaft of a balloon

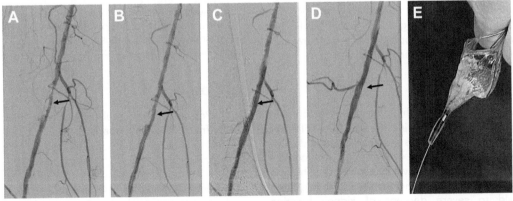

Fig. 3. (A), Lower extremity angiogram revealing severe (90%) calcific, occlusive plaque in the P2 segment of the popliteal artery (arrow); (B) Orbital atherectomy was used with the mild improvement of stenosis; (C), 6.0 × 60 mm Shockwave balloon was used for multiple treatments with the marked improvement of stenosis; (D), Further treatment with a 5.0 × 80 mm drug-coated balloon resulted in successful revascularization; (E), Retrieved filter with calcific debris in the basket.

angioplasty catheter can deliver localized pulsatile acoustic pressure waves circumferentially to modify vascular calcium.[45] In comparison with routine atherectomy and balloon angioplasty, IVL offers several advantages. IVL uses acoustic shockwaves delivered through a semicompliant balloon inflated to only 4 atm, thus avoiding high-pressure inflation and consequent potential barotrauma observed with conventional non-compliant balloons (**Fig. 2**). Atherectomy generates microparticulate debris that may embolize causing resultant tissue ischemia. IVL induces multiple regions of fracture of the plaque without actual VC removal from the vessel architecture. In addition, atheroablative technologies have the potential to only target superficial calcium with possible thermal and vascular complications of the target vessels. Alternatively, IVL fractures both superficial and deep calcium and minimizes the risk for vascular complications or thermal injury (**Fig. 3**).[45] In addition to previous cadaveric studies that used IVL, Disrupt CAD I (Shockwave Coronary Rx Lithoplasty Study), Disrupt CAD II (Shockwave Coronary Lithoplasty Study), and Disrupt CAD III (Disrupt CAD III With the Shockwave Coronary IVL System) optical coherence tomographic (OCT) sub-studies[46–48] and Disrupt PAD II OCT sub analyses[49] demonstrated superficial and deep calcium fractures on CT and histopathological specimens. A few observations made in previous studies include increase luminal gain due to superficial, deep, circumferential, and longitudinal calcium fractures, and improved vessel compliance with appropriate stent expansion. Thus, it was demonstrated that there was an increase in arterial luminal area following IVL without significant barotrauma. Multiple trials report the safety and effectiveness of IVL involving both severely calcified coronary and peripheral artery disease.[45,50,51] According to Disrupt PAD III, IVL was superior to angioplasty for procedural success and primary patency at 1 year.[52]

SUMMARY

CKD is associated with a plethora of factors that contribute to CVD including PAD. Different manifestations such as atherosclerosis and calcifications may have overlapping yet distinct mechanisms. The prevalence of PAD is high in patients with CKD and increases moving from mild to severe degrees of kidney function impairment. Percutaneous revascularization with new emerging technologies such as IVL has been shown to safely treat severe calcific plaque in patients with CKD with minimal complications. Although acute outcomes following IVL in severely calcified lesions are promising, longer term follow-up is required. As there are advances in endovascular therapy, large, randomized studies are needed to refine risk stratification and elucidate optimal treatment strategies for patients with CKD and PAD.

CLINICS CARE POINTS

- The risk of peripheral arterial disease (PAD) and chronic limb ischemia (CLI) is increased in patients with chronic kidney disease (CKD) and is related to the degree of kidney function impairment.
- CKD and albuminuria are independent risk factors of vascular calcification that affect treatment strategies and clinical outcomes. Intimal and medial vascular calcification occur through the myriad of pathways such as altered bone-mineral hemostasis, uremia, and inflammation in patients with CKD.
- Ankle-brachial index is considered the first line to detect PAD; however, medial calcification may pose falsely elevated values. Toe brachial index (TBI), ≤0.70 is accepted as a diagnostic value in patients with medial calcification.
- Invasive angiography is the gold standard test to define anatomy and plan for intervention.
- Revascularization, percutaneous or surgical, is indicated in patients with CKD and severe PAD with symptomatic and limiting claudication to improve symptomatology and prognosis in terms of amputation rate and mortality.
- New emerging technologies such as intravascular lithotripsy have been shown to effectively treat calcific plaque while minimizing complications.

DISCLOSURE

Dr A. Prasad reports receiving speaking honorarium from Shockwave medical.

REFERENCES

1. Creager MA. The crisis of vascular disease and the journey to vascular health. Circulation 2016;133: 2593–8.
2. Gerhard-Herman MD, Gornik HL, Barrett C, et al. 2016 AHA/ACC guideline on the management of patients with lower extremity peripheral artery

disease: executive summary: a report of the American college of cardiology/American heart association task force on clinical practice guidelines. Circulation 2017;135:e686–725.

3. Rocha-Singh KJ, Zeller T, Jaff MR. Peripheral arterial calcification: Prevalence, mechanism, detection, and clinical implications. Catheter Cardiovasc Interv 2014;83:E212–20.

4. Levey AS, Coresh J. Chronic kidney disease. Lancet (London, England) 2012;379:165–80.

5. Moe SM, Chen NX. Pathophysiology of vascular calcification in chronic kidney disease. Circ Res 2004;95:560–7.

6. Selvin E, Erlinger TP. Prevalence of and risk factors for peripheral arterial disease in the United States: results from the National Health and Nutrition Examination Survey, 1999-2000. Circulation 2004;110:738–43.

7. Matsushita K, Ballew SH, Coresh J, et al. Measures of chronic kidney disease and risk of incident peripheral artery disease: a collaborative meta-analysis of individual participant data. Lancet Diabetes Endocrinol 2017;5:718–28.

8. Provenzano M, Coppolino G, De Nicola L, et al. Unraveling cardiovascular risk in renal patients: a new take on old tale. Front Cell Dev Biol 2019;7:2–8.

9. Perticone M, Maio R, Sciacqua A, et al. Serum phosphorus levels are associated with endothelial dysfunction in hypertensive patients. Nutr Metab Cardiovasc Dis 2016;26:683–8.

10. Theilade S, Lajer M, Jorsal A, et al. Arterial stiffness and endothelial dysfunction independently and synergistically predict cardiovascular and renal outcome in patients with type 1 diabetes. Diabet Med 2012;29:990–4.

11. Huang MJ, Wei RB, Zhao J, et al. Albuminuria and endothelial dysfunction in patients with non-diabetic chronic kidney disease. Med Sci Mon Int Med J Exp Clin Res 2017;23:4447–53.

12. Hayden MR, Tyagi SC, Kolb L, et al. Vascular ossification-calcification in metabolic syndrome, type 2 diabetes mellitus, chronic kidney disease, and calciphylaxis-calcific uremic arteriolopathy: the emerging role of sodium thiosulfate. Cardiovasc Diabetol 2005;4:4.

13. Karwowski W, Naumnik B, Szczepański M, et al. The mechanism of vascular calcification - a systematic review. Med Sci Mon Int Med J Exp Clin Res 2012;18:Ra1–11.

14. Schlieper G, Schurgers L, Brandenburg V, et al. Vascular calcification in chronic kidney disease: an update. Nephrol Dial Transplant 2016;31:31–9.

15. Ketteler M, Schlieper G, Floege J. Calcification and cardiovascular health. Hypertension 2006;47:1027–34.

16. Yuen NK, Ananthakrishnan S, Campbell MJ. Hyperparathyroidism of renal disease. Perm J 2016;20:15–127.

17. Neven E, D'Haese PC. Vascular calcification in chronic renal failure. Circ Res 2011;108:249–64.

18. Chertow GM, Raggi P, Chasan-Taber S, et al. Determinants of progressive vascular calcification in haemodialysis patients. Nephrol Dial Transplant 2004;19:1489–96.

19. Galassi A, Spiegel DM, Bellasi A, et al. Accelerated vascular calcification and relative hypoparathyroidism in incident haemodialysis diabetic patients receiving calcium binders. Nephrol Dial Transplant 2006;21:3215–22.

20. Moe SM, Reslerova M, Ketteler M, et al. Role of calcification inhibitors in the pathogenesis of vascular calcification in chronic kidney disease (CKD). Kidney Int 2005;67:2295–304.

21. O'Neill WC, Sigrist MK, McIntyre CW. Plasma pyrophosphate and vascular calcification in chronic kidney disease. Nephrol Dial Transplant 2010;25:187–91.

22. Brandenburg VM, Sinha S, Specht P, et al. Calcific uraemic arteriolopathy: a rare disease with a potentially high impact on chronic kidney disease–mineral and bone disorder. Pediatr Nephrol 2014;29:2289–98.

23. Criqui MH, Matsushita K, Aboyans V, et al. Lower extremity peripheral artery disease: contemporary epidemiology, management gaps, and future directions: a scientific statement from the American Heart association. Circulation 2021;144:e171–91.

24. Teraa M, Conte MS, Moll FL, et al. Critical limb ischemia: current trends and future directions. J Am Heart Assoc 2016;5:e002938.

25. Hirsch AT, Criqui MH, Treat-Jacobson D, et al. Peripheral arterial disease detection, awareness, and treatment in primary care. JAMA 2001;286:1317–24.

26. Lijmer JG, Hunink MGM, van den Dungen JJAM, et al. ROC analysis of noninvasive tests for peripheral arterial disease. Ultrasound Med Biol 1996;22:391–8.

27. Aboyans V, Ricco J-B, Bartelink M, et al. ESC scientific document group. 2017 ESC guidelines on the diagnosis and treatment of peripheral arterial diseases, in collaboration with the European society for vascular surgery (ESVS): Document covering atherosclerotic disease of extracranial carotid and vertebral, mesenteric, renal, upper and lower extremity arteriesEndorsed by: the European stroke organization (ESO) The task force for the diagnosis and treatment of peripheral arterial diseases of the European society of cardiology (ESC) and of the European society for vascular surgery (ESVS). Eur Heart J 2018;39:763–816.

28. AbuRahma AF, Adams E, AbuRahma J, et al. Critical analysis and limitations of resting ankle-brachial index in the diagnosis of symptomatic peripheral arterial disease patients and the role of diabetes mellitus and chronic kidney disease. J Vasc Surg 2020;71:937–45.

29. Kamath TP, Prasad R, Allison MA, et al. Association of ankle-brachial and toe-brachial indexes with mortality in patients with CKD. Kidney Medicine 2020;2(1):68–75.

30. Buls N, de Brucker Y, Aerden D, et al. Improving the diagnosis of peripheral arterial disease in below-the-knee arteries by adding time-resolved CT scan series to conventional run-off CT angiography. First experience with a 256-slice CT scanner. Eur J Radiol 2019;110:136–41.

31. Weinreb JC, Rodby RA, Yee J, et al. Use of intravenous gadolinium-based contrast media in patients with kidney disease: consensus statements from the American college of radiology and the national kidney foundation. Radiology 2021;298:28–35.

32. Ghumman SS, Weinerman J, Khan A, et al. Contrast induced-acute kidney injury following peripheral angiography with carbon dioxide versus iodinated contrast media: a meta-analysis and systematic review of current literature. Catheter Cardiovasc Interv 2017;90:437–48.

33. Kereiakes Dean J, Virmani R, Hokama Jason Y, et al. Principles of intravascular lithotripsy for calcific plaque modification. JACC Cardiovasc Interv 2021;14:1275–92.

34. De Vriese AS, Caluwé R, Pyfferoen L, et al. Multicenter randomized controlled trial of vitamin K Antagonist Replacement by Rivaroxaban with or without Vitamin K2 in hemodialysis patients with atrial fibrillation: the valkyrie study. J Am Soc Nephrol : JASN (J Am Soc Nephrol) 2020;31:186–96.

35. Bressendorff I, Hansen D, Schou M, et al. The effect of magnesium supplementation on vascular calcification in CKD: a randomized clinical trial (MAGiCAL-CKD). J Am Soc Nephrol : JASN (J Am Soc Nephrol) 2023;34:886–94.

36. Djuric P, Dimkovic N, Schlieper G, et al. Sodium thiosulphate and progression of vascular calcification in end-stage renal disease patients: a double-blind, randomized, placebo-controlled study. Nephrol Dial Transplant 2020;35:162–9.

37. Agarwal S, Sud K, Shishehbor MH. Nationwide trends of hospital admission and outcomes among critical limb ischemia patients: from 2003–2011. J Am Coll Cardiol 2016;67:1901–13.

38. Garimella PS, Balakrishnan P, Correa A, et al. Nationwide trends in hospital outcomes and utilization after lower limb revascularization in patients on hemodialysis. JACC Cardiovasc Interv 2017;10:2101–10.

39. Farber A, Menard MT, Conte MS, et al. Surgery or endovascular therapy for chronic limb-threatening ischemia. N Engl J Med 2022;387:2305–16.

40. Katsanos K, Spiliopoulos S, Reppas L, et al. Debulking atherectomy in the peripheral arteries: is there a role and what is the evidence? Cardiovasc Intervent Radiol 2017;40:964–77.

41. Mittleider D, Russell E. Peripheral atherectomy: applications and techniques. Tech Vasc Interv Radiol 2016;19:123–35.

42. Diamantopoulos A, Katsanos K. Atherectomy of the femoropopliteal artery: a systematic review and meta-analysis of randomized controlled trials. J Cardiovasc Surg 2014;55:655–65.

43. Shammas NW, Coiner D, Shammas GA, et al. Percutaneous lower-extremity arterial interventions with primary balloon angioplasty versus Silverhawk atherectomy and adjunctive balloon angioplasty: randomized trial. J Vasc Interv Radiol 2011;22:1223–8.

44. Shammas NW, Lam R, Mustapha J, et al. Comparison of orbital atherectomy plus balloon angioplasty vs. balloon angioplasty alone in patients with critical limb ischemia: results of the CALCIUM 360 randomized pilot trial. J Endovasc Ther 2012;19:480–8.

45. Tepe G, Brodmann M, Werner M, et al. Intravascular lithotripsy for peripheral artery calcification. JACC Cardiovasc Interv 2021;14:1352–61.

46. Kereiakes Dean J, Di Mario C, Riley Robert F, et al. Intravascular lithotripsy for treatment of calcified coronary lesions. JACC Cardiovasc Interv 2021;14:1337–48.

47. Ali ZA, Nef H, Escaned J, et al. Safety and effectiveness of coronary intravascular lithotripsy for treatment of severely calcified coronary stenoses: the disrupt CAD II study. Circulation: Cardiovascular Interventions 2019;12:e008434.

48. Madhavan MV, Shahim B, Mena-Hurtado C, et al. Efficacy and safety of intravascular lithotripsy for the treatment of peripheral arterial disease: an individual patient-level pooled data analysis. Catheter Cardiovasc Interv 2020;95:959–68.

49. Holden A. Safety and performance of the Shockwave Lithoplasty System in treating calcified peripheral vascular lesions: intravascular OCT analysis. Leipzig, Germany: LINC; 2018.

50. Brodmann M, Werner M, Brinton TJ, et al. Safety and performance of lithoplasty for treatment of calcified peripheral artery lesions. J Am Coll Cardiol 2017;70:908–10.

51. Brodmann M, Werner M, Holden A, et al. Primary outcomes and mechanism of action of intravascular lithotripsy in calcified, femoropopliteal lesions: results of Disrupt PAD II. Catheter Cardiovasc Interv 2019;93:335–42.

52. Tepe G, Brodmann M, Bachinsky W, et al. Intravascular lithotripsy for peripheral artery calcification: mid-term outcomes from the randomized disrupt PAD III trial. Journal of the Society for Cardiovascular Angiography & Interventions 2022;1:2–7.

Implications of Renal Disease in Patients Undergoing Structural Interventions

Adam Pampori, MD, Shashank Shekhar, MD,
Samir R. Kapadia, MD*

KEYWORDS

- Percutaneous structural interventions • Chronic kidney disease • End-stage renal disease
- Acute kidney injury • TAVR • TEER

KEY POINTS

- Patients with CKD and ESRD represent a population with high surgical risk and high prevalence of severe VHD.
- AKI remains a significant perioperative complication that is predictive of poor outcomes; stringent protocols and a team-based approach are needed to avoid this complication.
- Renal disease has a significant impact on outcomes of these percutaneous structural interventions.

INTRODUCTION

Percutaneous structural interventions have revolutionized the world of cardiology in the last two decades. Even though valvulopathy has significant morbidity, mortality, and reduced quality of life, previously, treatment was limited to high-risk cardiac surgery, and many patients were often not offered treatment because of real or perceived risks.[1,2] Symptomatic aortic stenosis (AS) is associated with high mortality when untreated,[3,4] and although surgical aortic valve replacement (SAVR) was previously the gold standard, transcatheter aortic valve replacement (TAVR) has emerged as a treatment of choice in patients with severe AS; in fact, the American College of Cardiology and American Heart Association 2020 guidelines recommend TAVR for all symptomatic patients at high surgical risk or when older than 80 years,[5] with further trials under way for intermediate- and low-risk patients. Similarly, transcatheter edge-to-edge mitral valve repair (TEER) has emerged as a technique that can reduce symptoms, improve functional capacity, and improve the quality of life in patients with mitral regurgitation (MR).[6–9]

The presence of chronic kidney disease (CKD)/ end-stage renal disease (ESRD) and occurrence of acute kidney injury (AKI) play an important role in the morbidity and mortality associated with structural heart diseases. Moreover, these diseases can have strong impacts on short- and long-term outcomes after structural interventions. In this review, we explore the current state of the art in acute kidney disease and CKD, major risk factors that impact outcomes, and techniques to minimize risks and poor outcomes.

ACUTE KIDNEY INJURY

Rapid loss of kidney function within hours to days with resultant impairment of electrolytes, volume, and waste excretion is defined as AKI. AKI is a common complication associated with

Department of Cardiovascular Medicine, Heart and Vascular Institute, Cleveland Clinic, 9500 Euclid Avenue, J2-3, Cleveland, OH 44195, USA
* Corresponding author.
E-mail address: kapadis@ccf.org
Twitter: tavrkapadia (S.R.K.)

Intervent Cardiol Clin 12 (2023) 539–554
https://doi.org/10.1016/j.iccl.2023.06.002

transcatheter cardiac procedures and is associated with poor prognosis. The criteria used to define AKI has varied over time. Since 2012, trials have mostly adopted the standardized AKI definition from the Valve Academic Research Consortium-2 (VARC-2), a group founded in 2010 to standardize end points and definitions for TAVR and SAVR trials.[10] This definition is based on the KDIGO (Kidney Disease: Improving Global Outcomes) definition used by many in the nephrology community.[11,12] Recently, the VARC-3 definitions (Table 1) were published with changes to these criteria in 2021.[13] Urine output was removed because of challenges in its use in daily practice[14,15]; instead, the guidelines recommend considering the usage of urine output criteria in the setting of dedicated AKI studies. Also, a fourth stage was added: requirement for new renal-replacement therapy (temporary or permanent) in VARC-3.

Risk Factors and Pathophysiology

The pathogenesis of AKI poststructural intervention is multifactorial, including a combination of preprocedure, intraprocedure, and postprocedure factors (Table 2). These factors likely create a combination of prerenal azotemia and direct nephrotoxic effects, leading to renal ischemia and acute tubular necrosis. These include the use of nephrotoxic agents, atherosclerotic emboli, intraprocedure hypotension, ischemia-reperfusion injury, inflammatory response, and red blood cell (RBC) transfusions.

Preprocedural factors generally consist of patient comorbidities. (1) Patients at higher operative risk (as measured by calculators, such as the Society of Thoracic Surgeons or the EuroSCORE II) had higher AKI rates in multiple studies, likely reflecting the baseline poor health status of those patients.[16–19] (2) CKD at baseline is one of the strongest predictors of postprocedure AKI in multiple studies.[17,18,20–24] In an analysis of the Nationwide Inpatient Sample (NIS), CKD predicted AKI with an odds ratio (OR) of 3.52 (95% confidence interval [CI], 3.40–3.64),[21] whereas a meta-analysis by Wang and colleagues[17] with 661 post-TAVR patients with AKI and 2012 control subjects using a multivariate analysis demonstrated an OR of 2.81 (95% CI, 1.96–4.03). Because of their baseline renal dysfunction, this population likely has lower physiologic reserve and deficient autoregulatory mechanisms to handle periprocedural renal stresses, and therefore are more sensitive to renal injury than patients without baseline CKD. (3) Chronic obstructive pulmonary disease and respiratory failure have been shown to predict AKI post-TAVR,[18,21,22,25] likely via increased hypoxia and arterial carbon dioxide levels, leading to reduced renal blood flow, glomerular filtration, and neurohormonal activation.[18,26] (4) In some studies, prior cardiovascular diseases and metabolic syndrome also predict AKI. For instance, a history of hypertension, diabetes, or stroke were predictive of the development of AKI in an analysis from the NIS database.[21] Hypertension, diabetes, and stroke are all strongly associated with macrovascular and microvascular complications throughout the body, including the kidneys. These conditions likely increase the susceptibility of the kidneys to renal hypoperfusion, which makes these patients more susceptible to AKI. (5) A history of heart failure and atrial fibrillation have been shown to be predictive of AKI.[17,21,27] New York Heart Association class IV heart failure was strongly associated with post-TAVR AKI in a meta-analysis by Wang and colleagues[17] (OR, 7.77; 95% CI, 3.87–15.85). Being sensitive to volume status, maintaining euvolemia in these patients is paramount to their care. This is likely attributable to the vulnerability of patients with advanced heart failure to cardiorenal syndrome.[28] (6) Generalized atherosclerosis and peripheral vascular disease (PVD) are common comorbidities in patients requiring structural

Table 1	
VARC-3 (Valve Academic Research Consortium-3) criteria for AKI	
Stage 1	Increase in serum creatinine to 150%–199% (1.5–1.99 × increase compared with baseline) within 7 days OR Increase of ≥0.3 mg/dL (≥26.4 mmol/L) within 48 h of the index procedure
Stage 2	Increase in serum creatinine to 200%–300% (2.0–3.0 × increase compared with baseline) within 7 days
Stage 3	Increase in serum creatinine to >300% (>3 × increase compared with baseline) OR serum creatinine of ≥4.0 mg/dL (≥354 mmol/L) with an acute increase of at least 0.5 mg/dL (44 mmol/L)
Stage 4	AKI requiring new temporary or permanent renal-replacement therapy

Urine output may be considered in the context of dedicated AKI studies.

Table 2
Factors associated with AKI following TAVR

Preprocedure Factors	Intraprocedure Factors	Postprocedure Factors
• Age • Preexisting kidney disease • Recent contrast exposure • Heart failure • Peripheral artery disease • Diabetes • Hypertension • Prior stroke • Anemia	• Hypotension (most often caused by rapid ventricular pacing) • Bleeding and blood transfusion requirement • Embolic events • Transapical approach • Complicated or prolonged cases requiring mechanical circulatory support • Ischemia-reperfusion injury • Inflammatory response • General anesthesia	• Need for vasoconstricting agents • Use of nephrotoxins • Decreased heart function/heart failure • Grade of aortic regurgitation after the procedure

interventions; therefore, manipulation of the aorta with large-lumen catheters carries a risk of cholesterol embolism, including embolization to the kidneys leading to AKI.[14,18,29–35] One study using computed tomographic (CT) imaging to evaluate aortic suprarenal atherosclerosis demonstrated that atheroma burden directly correlated with AKI.[36] PVD has been shown in multiple studies to be an independent risk factor for AKI post-TAVR.[23,25,37–39] In TAVR, scraping of aortic plaques by catheters has been observed in most subjects,[33,34] leading to the advent of the use of cerebral embolic protection devices to protect from neurologic complications[40] with mixed results.[34,41]

Procedural characteristics, such as the use of transapical approach over transfemoral approach, further increase the risk of embolization and AKI, even though the former usually requires lesser contrast media (CM) in comparison with the latter.[16,42–44] This may be caused by the need for general anesthesia with transapical approach, which increases the risk for hypotension and poor renal blood flow. Another hypothesis relates to an inflammatory reaction because of surgical trauma.[45] Regardless of the trigger, studies consistently show reduced mortality and kidney injury with transfemoral approach; therefore, transfemoral approach is generally preferred unless there is advanced arterial occlusive disease limiting femoral access.[32,42,46] Kidneys have the highest tissue perfusion rate in relation to organ weight in the body, thus making them particularly susceptible to hemodynamic injury. Decreased blood flow to the kidneys is likely a major cause for postprocedural AKI and is caused by several potential etiologies. In TAVR, rapid ventricular pacing during balloon valvuloplasty and valve implantation leading to brief periods of inadequate cardiac filling time may cause brief episodes of hypotension and decreased renal blood flow.[18,29,47–49]

Postprocedural paravalvular regurgitation may lead to reduced overall effective cardiac output and thus, reduced renal blood flow.[50–53] Inotropic support and vasoconstrictors are well-established to vasoconstrict renal arterioles and may lead to AKI, although this must be balanced with maintaining systemic perfusion.[54,55] After recovery from an initial hemodynamic insult, ischemia-reperfusion injury may occur, further exacerbating AKI.[56]

Bleeding also leads to hypotension and decreased blood flow, and the need for blood transfusion has been shown to be a strong independent predictor for AKI.[31] Anemia itself can contribute to kidney injury via reduced renal oxygen delivery.[57] RBCs serve an important function as antioxidants, and therefore anemia may worsen oxidative stress.[58] During storage before transfusion, RBCs undergo structural changes; they can lose their deformability, undergo adenosine triphosphate and 2,3-diphosphoglycerate depletion, accumulate proinflammatory molecules, and increase procoagulant lipids.[58–60] One study showed a three-fold increase in post-TAVR AKI in patients who received RBC transfusions,[18] which correlates with several other studies.[16,19,38]

CM is well established as a cause of AKI, which generally occurs within days after the procedure,[61] although more recent data suggest that the risk may be overestimated.[62–65] One study found the volume of CM used multiplied by the serum creatinine and divided by body weight greater than 2.99 predicted AKI with a sensitivity of 85.7% and specificity of 90.4%.[66] Another study suggested that calculating the ratio of CM volume divided by glomerular filtration rate (GFR) less than 3.9 predicted AKI with 71% sensitivity and 80% specificity.[67] CM is thought to cause AKI via multiple possible direct or indirect mechanisms. The pathogenesis of contrast-associated nephropathy is discussed in detail in another chapter.

Prevention of Acute Kidney Injury in Structural Interventions

Standard techniques to minimize postprocedural AKI are aimed at reducing impairment of renal blood flow, minimizing use of nephrotoxic medications (eg, contrast, vasoconstrictors), and maximizing cardiac output (by optimizing procedural result), although there are no specific trials regarding these measures in post-TAVR or post-TEER AKI.[29,68] Box 1 provides a list of recommended techniques.

A multidisciplinary team approach should be used when managing patients with CKD and severe valvular heart disease (VHD). The team should include a renal physician, with a goal of optimizing predisposing factors, maintaining euvolemic status, and discontinuing nephrotoxic medications before TAVR. Contrast dosage should be minimized, and low-osmolar contrast agents' usage may reduce AKI rates.

Multiple studies aimed at identifying interventions to prevent contrast-induced AKI have shown mixed results with the exception of minimizing contrast volume and optimizing hydration[69]; this is discussed in detail in (see Chaudhary and Kashani's article, "Acute Kidney Injury Management Strategies Peri-Cardiovascular Interventions," in this issue), (see Solomon's article, "Hydration to Prevent Contrast-Associated Acute Kidney Injury in Patients Undergoing Cardiac Angiography," in this issue).

Box 1
Methods to reduce risk of acute kidney injury after transcatheter procedures

- Use a team-based approach, including a nephrologist, to optimize preprocedure factors
- Gain experience; if low-volume, refer patients to a high-volume center
- Minimize contrast use, prefer low- or iso-osmolar agents
- Optimize hydration
- Minimize rapid ventricular pacing
- Avoid intraoperative hypotension
- Minimize perioperative inotropes/vasoconstrictors using goal-directed therapy
- Minimize postoperative paravalvular regurgitation
- Avoid bleeding and minimize use of blood transfusions
- Prefer a transfemoral over transapical approach

Transcatheter Aortic Valve Replacement

AKI is a complication seen in post-TAVR patients that was identified as one of the most common complications in the landmark Placement of AoRTic TraNscathetER Valve (PARTNER) trials.[70–73] Reported incidence of AKI after TAVR varies from 0.6% to 57%.[14,15,18,32,36,67,70–80] Part of this wide range is likely attributable to the variation in definitions and observation timelines (ie, some used 72 hours vs 7 days). Other explanations for this wide range include different valve prostheses, varying sample sizes, patient populations, varying techniques, center experience, and volume of CM used. Because techniques, operator experience, and valve technology have improved significantly over the past decade, earlier studies are likely not representative of contemporary outcomes. A summary of AKI rates in major trials is reported in Fig. 1.

Post-TAVR AKI is independently associated with a five- to eight-fold increase in 30-day mortality, at least a three-fold increase in 1-year mortality, longer hospital stays, and greater intensive care use.[32,37,74,81–83] Incidence of long-term hemodialysis is 21%.[31,46,74] An analysis from the NIS including 173,760 weighted hospitalizations demonstrated that no-AKI in comparison with patients with AKI post-TAVR were 10 times less likely to have in-hospital mortality (0.8% mortality in no-AKI vs 8% mortality in patients with AKI; $P < .01$).[21] Post-TAVR AKI may also be associated with progression of CKD; a cohort study by Witberg and colleagues[84] demonstrated that patients with AKI post-TAVR were more likely to have worse CKD at the 2-year follow-up, and in the same study those without AKI were more likely to have improved CKD. Major risk factors associated with post-TAVR AKI, and the pathophysiology of these risk factors is reviewed in detail previously.

Compared with surgical aortic valve replacement

As experience and techniques have advanced, TAVR offers several advantages over SAVR with respect to AKI risk, such as no need for general anesthesia or cardiopulmonary bypass, reduced risk of bleeding and transfusion, advances in three-dimensional echocardiography have reduced contrast usage, advances in techniques have led to lower paravalvular regurgitation, leading to better renal perfusion and often improvement in baseline kidney function. Although the early, pivotal PARTNER 1 trial showed no difference in AKI in SAVR versus TAVR, since then most trials demonstrated a lower risk of periprocedural AKI in TAVR

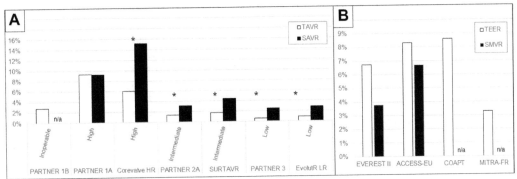

Fig. 1. (A) Rates of perioperative acute kidney injury in major TAVR trials compared with SAVR.[70–73,78–80] Surgical risk of the patient population of the trial is indicated above the trial name. (B) Rates of perioperative acute kidney injury in major TEER trials compared with SMVR.[8,89–91] Asterisk denotes statistical significance by the trial definition. HR, high risk; LR, low risk; n/a, no surgical group in these trials; PARTNER, Placement of AoRTic TraNscathetER valves; SMVR surgical mitral valve replacement; SURTAVR, SURgical or transcatheter aortic valve replacement.

(Fig. 1A).[70–73,78–80] Several meta-analyses have confirmed this, even when stratified by surgical risk.[32,85–88] One meta-analysis also showed a lower incidence of dialysis-requiring AKI in TAVR patients at low to intermediate surgical risk, and noninferiority in the high-risk population.[88]

Transcatheter Edge-to-Edge Mitral Valve Repair

In comparison with TAVR, less is known about AKI after TEER. Although the incidence of AKI in major TEER trials ranged from 1.6% to 8.6% (see Fig. 1B),[8,89–91] more recent observational studies demonstrate an incidence of 15% to 29%.[92–95] This may be caused by differences in patient population selected for the trials compared with the clinical population. For example, in a pooled meta-analysis compared with TEER arm in EVEREST II, a larger proportion of patients had New York Heart Association functional class III/IV (86% vs 52%), diabetes (31% vs 8%), and functional MR (66% vs 27%).[89,94] TEER patients who developed AKI compared with patients without AKI had significantly higher 30-day mortality, 1-year mortality, increased length of stay, 30-day all-cause readmissions, and 30-day heart failure readmissions.[94,96]

TEER is generally guided by transesophageal echocardiogram and does not use nephrotoxic contrast, suggesting the role of other risk factors, such as the cause of AKI. The strongest predictors in a pooled meta-analysis of AKI post-TEER included CKD, history of chronic obstructive pulmonary disease, device failure (ie, residual MR of 2+), heart failure, diabetes, and the use of norepinephrine.[94,96] Additionally, general anesthesia, bleeding, anemia, and use of other nephrotoxic agents has also been implicated in post-TEER AKI.[92]

Techniques to prevent and minimize risk of AKI are similar to the TAVR recommendations (see **Box 1**), although no specific trials addressing AKI exist in the TEER population. Transcatheter mitral valve replacement (TMVR) via a transapical or transseptal approach is on the horizon with promising results, but no devices have yet been approved for clinical use and no reports of its impact on renal function yet exist.

Mitral Balloon Valvuloplasty

Rheumatic mitral stenosis (MS) has a significant prevalence worldwide, but decreased incidence and prevalence in industrialized countries.[97–99] The first-line treatment of MS is percutaneous balloon mitral valvuloplasty (PBMV).[100] Off-label use of PBMV for calcific MS has increased over time in the United States likely because of higher rates of calcific valve disease in the aging population.[98] The reported incidence of AKI doubled from 5% to 10% from 2008 to 2018 in a study from the NIS (n = 3980).[101] Because PBMV does not require contrast, other mechanisms must be at play. PBMV hospitalizations decreased by 65% over the same period, suggesting that operator experience may be a factor. Rates of hypertension, diabetes, CKD, and heart failure have also increased, suggesting poor physiologic reserve and increased susceptibility of the population to AKI. More research is needed in this area.

CHRONIC KIDNEY DISEASE AND END-STAGE RENAL DISEASE

There is a high prevalence of calcific VHD in patients with renal dysfunction. Mortality rates at 5 years for these patients is twice as high compared with patients without renal dysfunction, even if valvular dysfunction is mild.[102] However, these patients often have multiple comorbidities and are at high risk for open cardiac surgery, making percutaneous valve interventions an attractive alternative.[25,103,104]

Epidemiology

Valvular calcification is directly correlated with decreasing estimated GFR.[105,106] On echocardiography, valvular calcification is seen in around 35% to 40% of patients with ESRD,[107,108] but only in 7.4% of patients with kidney transplantation,[109] although this could be a selection bias because transplant candidates tend to be healthier. A review of renal transplant trials by Cianciolo and colleagues[110] suggests that renal transplant may impede progression of valvular calcification but does not reverse it. In this population, AS is the most common VHD, and progresses twice as fast in patients with CKD.[106,111] Histologically, the prevalence of vascular calcification in radial arteries was 45-fold greater in patients with CKD.[112] Predictors of aortic valve calcification include age, malnutrition, inflammation, phosphate levels, calcium-phosphorous product, vitamin D levels, and duration of dialysis.[113–115]

Pathophysiology

VHD in CKD is multifactorial, caused by an imbalance of calcification promoters (calcium and phosphate) and inhibitors (matrix Gla protein and fetuin-A).[116] Renal dysfunction leads to failure of kidneys to convert enough vitamin D to its active form (1,25-dihydroxycholecalciferol) along with inadequate phosphate excretion. Elevated phosphorus levels facilitate the formation of insoluble calcium-phosphate leading to calcium deposition and hypocalcemia, resulting in secondary hyperparathyroidism.[117] Moreover, in response to high serum phosphate and parathyroid hormone, osteoblasts produce fibroblast growth factor-23, which inhibits conversion of vitamin D to its active form and elevated fibroblast growth factor-23 levels have been proposed as one of the mediators of calcification in CKD.[118] Additionally, elevated uremic toxins because of renal failure drive inflammatory biomarkers and combine to trigger valvular calcification.[116] Vitamin K antagonists, such as warfarin, are linked to valve calcification likely via interference with matrix Gla protein, which is a vitamin K–dependent protein.[119,120] This mechanism raised the hypothesis that repletion with vitamin K may reduce progression of valvular calcification; however, subsequent trials have been unsuccessful in demonstrating the same.[121]

Hemodynamically, calcification of vessels contributes to increased pulse wave velocity, earlier reflection of the pulse wave, and increased cardiac afterload, resulting in left ventricular hypertrophy, increased shear stress, and progression of aortic valve calcification. AS may also reduce cardiac output and cause cardiorenal syndrome, thereby exacerbating renal dysfunction. Additionally, arteriovenous fistulas used for dialysis access may lead to high output heart failure, and cardiac chamber enlargement, which can cause functional mitral and tricuspid regurgitation.[122,123] The link between arteriovenous fistulas and progression of valve calcification is unclear. Patients with ESRD have extensive mitral annular calcification (MAC), which has a similar pathophysiology to aortic valve calcification.[124–126] Congenital conditions, such as bicuspid aortic valves, also increase shear stress on the valve and accelerate calcification.[127] As a result of these changes, these patients are prone to endocarditis and atrial arrhythmias, both of which are associated with a high mortality rate.[128]

CKD is an established risk factor for bioprosthetic valve failure via the previously mentioned mechanisms. The calcification inherent in cardiac tissue of patients with CKD and ESRD creates a hostile landing zone for prosthetic valves. The biochemical insults created by CKD are not changed by valve replacement, and can lead to structural valve deterioration, including intrinsic deterioration of bioprosthetic leaflets or support structure because of thickening, calcification, tearing, or disruption of the prosthesis leading to hemodynamic failure, valve thrombosis, or infective endocarditis.[129]

Diagnostic Considerations

The cornerstone of assessment of VHD is echocardiography. The diagnosis and evaluation of VHD in patients with CKD is confounded by anemia, frailty, hypertension, and volume status, and thus, echocardiography is best performed when patient is euvolemic and with good blood pressure control, that is, after dialysis. Echocardiogram is limited by large body habitus, leading to suboptimal windows. Septal hypertrophy is common in patients with CKD, which can make calculation of left ventricular outflow tract (LVOT) area difficult. Arteriovenous fistulas can lead to a high output state and cause overestimation of transvalvular gradients; to mitigate this, temporary arteriovenous compression is used.[130] In patients with paradoxic low-flow/low-gradient severe AS, a dimensionless severity index less than 0.25 indicates severe AS and should be used more often than aortic valve area because it is less variable and more reproducible, and predicts prognosis.[131–133]

Cardiac CT is a noninvasive modality that has transformed the preoperative assessment of severe AS. It provides information critical to preoperative planning and feasibility assessment of TAVR, including annulus measurement, calcium distribution, coronary ostia, and vascular anatomy. An aortic valve calcium score greater than or equal to 2000 Agatston units in men or greater than or equal to 1200 in women is diagnostic of severe AS.[134]

Because patients with CKD are particularly susceptible to contrast nephropathy, other alternatives may also be considered. Low contrast cardiac CT protocols have been developed.[135] Transesophageal echocardiogram may be used as an alternative.[136] Cardiac MRI may be used instead of cardiac CT because it can quantitatively assess aortic valve function and provides all measurements needed for the procedure, although it is limited with regard to evaluation of calcification.[137] Gadolinium-based contrast used in cardiac MRI is significantly less nephrotoxic than iodine-based contrast used in CT,[138] and late enhancement allows for evaluation of macroscopic fibrosis in AS. Cardiac MRI is far less used than cardiac CT, likely because it is technically more complex, requires a longer study time, and a higher degree of patient cooperation.[139]

Pharmacologic Options

To date, no effective pharmacologic options exist to reverse valve calcification in patients with CKD or ESRD. Data suggesting lipid accumulation in calcified valves prompted trials of cholesterol-lowering therapies. However, the Simvastatin and Ezetimibe in Aortic Stenosis trial, the largest trial to date, showed no effects on AS progression.[140] Renin-angiotensin-aldosterone system inhibitors showed some promise in animal studies but had contradictory impact in retrospective studies.[141,142] Given the effect of vitamin K antagonists on valve calcification, vitamin K supplementation was hypothesized to reduce progression of valvular calcification; trials have, however, been unsuccessful.[121] Phosphate-lowering therapies had mixed results.[143,144] Medications targeting osteoporosis were recently evaluated for AS with negative results.[145] Given the lack of proven pharmacologic options, valve replacement is the mainstay therapy for patients with severe AS.

Transcatheter Aortic Valve Replacement

The most common VHD in individuals with ESRD and CKD is aortic valve disease.[146] The mortality of patients on dialysis after SAVR is nearly 20%, and rises to 50% in elderly dialysis patients.[147–149] TAVR provides an attractive minimally invasive alternative and has quickly become the procedure of choice in this high-risk population. Until recently, TAVR trials excluded patients with advanced CKD or ESRD, but several trials including these patients have recently been published.

A 5-year pooled outcomes analysis of PARTNER 2A and SAPIEN 3 registries of patients with moderate to severe CKD (estimated GFR, <60 mL/min/m^2) did not demonstrate a statistically significant difference between TAVR and SAVR for death alone or the composite outcome of death, stroke, rehospitalization, and new dialysis requirement. However, perioperative AKI was more than twice as likely with SAVR (10.3% vs 26.3%; $P < .001$).[150] Another analysis of 5190 patients from the PARTNER 1, 2, and PARTNER 2 S3 trials of patients with CKD showed that CKD stage after TAVR either improved or was unchanged, suggesting that AS maybe contributory to cardiorenal syndrome in these patients, which improves with TAVR.[151]

The largest meta-analysis to date of TAVR in patients with CKD analyzed 133,624 patients and demonstrated higher mortality at 30-day, 1-year, and 2-year follow-up in patients with CKD compared with those without, and mortality correlated with worsening severity of CKD.[152] CKD was associated with increased AKI (relative risk, 1.38; 95% CI, 1.16–1.63) and bleeding (relative risk, 1.33; 95% CI, 1.18–1.50), but not major vascular complications, stroke, or permanent pacemaker implantation. The largest study to date that compared TAVR outcomes between dialysis and nondialysis patients comes from the transcatheter valve therapies registry.[153] An analysis of 3000 dialysis patients found that these patients were younger, had higher Society of Thoracic Surgeons scores, were more likely to be African American, and more likely to have multiple comorbidities. This cohort also had a higher prevalence of MR, tricuspid regurgitation, and poor left ventricular systolic function. When they underwent TAVR, they were more likely to have lower use of the transfemoral approach, likely because of concomitant severe PVD. Dialysis patients experienced substantially higher in-hospital mortality (5.1% vs 3.4%; $P < .01$), 1-year mortality (relative risk, 1.28; 95% CI, 1.17–1.41), and higher rates of major bleeding and major vascular complications.

Patients with renal dysfunction likely have worse outcomes because of CKD-related platelet dysfunction, anemia of chronic disease,

PVD, diabetes, and frailty among other comorbidities. Mortality in patients with CKD has improved over time[154–158] likely because of improved operator expertise, center volumes, and device technology over time.

Patient selection is vital in this high-risk population. One study demonstrated a mortality rate of 71% in patients with advanced CKD with pre-existing atrial fibrillation and dialysis therapy at 1-year follow-up post-TAVR.[154] Other potential markers of futility include frailty, severe MR, severe pulmonary hypertension, and oxygen-dependent chronic respiratory failure.[159] Further research is needed to identify which patients with ESRD would benefit from TAVR.

Compared with surgical aortic valve replacement

However, it is important to view this in the context of the alternative: SAVR. In comparison with SAVR, TAVR avoids extracorporeal circulation, reduces risk of bleeding and transfusion, hypothermia, perioperative hypotension, non-pulsatile blood flow, euvolemic hemodilution, and ischemia-reperfusion injury.[74,160–162] A meta-analysis comparing 9619 patients with CKD undergoing TAVR versus SAVR demonstrated TAVR was associated with lower risk of early all-cause mortality (6.1% vs 10.2%; OR, 0.71; 95% CI, 0.37–0.75), stroke, transfusion, infection, AKI, and AKI requiring dialysis.[163] Similar outcomes were observed in another meta-analysis limited to patients with advanced CKD (stages 3–5).[164]

Transcatheter Mitral Valve Interventions
Transcatheter edge-to-edge mitral valve repair

CKD is frequently associated with MR, which may accelerate renal dysfunction by reducing stroke volume and increased pulmonary hypertension.[165] Surgical mitral valve intervention has a high mortality rate. The MitraClip has been proven to be an effective alternative for patients with MR at high risk for surgery[166] and avoids cardiopulmonary bypass, contrast, and other nephrotoxins, making it ideal for patients with CKD. Multiple studies demonstrate improvement in renal function in nearly one-third of cases,[165,167–170] although survival is lower compared with patients without CKD.[167,168,171] This improvement is most likely caused by improved stroke volume and cardiac output after repair, likely improving cardiorenal syndrome. It is unclear which patients would benefit from TEER, and further research in this area is needed.

Mitral annular calcification

MAC is common in patients with CKD and is characterized by fibrous, degenerative calcification.[105] MAC commonly leads to functional MS or mixed MS and MR. Patients with CKD or ESRD are often poor candidates for open cardiac surgery. Several devices for TMVR are on the horizon and may be a viable alternative for this population, although no studies currently exist in the CKD population. Common complications of TMVR include conduction defects, paravalvular regurgitation, aortic root injury, and left LVOT obstruction. LVOT obstruction is of particular concern because it is unpredictable and cataclysmic (1-month mortality hazard ratio, 3.16; 95% CI, 1.19–8.36). Severe MAC is associated with LVOT obstruction at rates of 54%, likely caused by a combination of MS, small left ventricular cavity, and intact anterior mitral leaflet. The aortomitral angle and implantation depth of the device are strong predictors of the degree of obstruction, but this risk is reduced by prophylactic alcohol septal ablation or laceration of the anterior mitral leaflet before device implantation if the neo-LVOT area is less than 1.7 cm², which is a strong predictor of obstruction.[172] All-cause mortality rates of 53.7% after 1-year post-TMVR have been reported.[173] Further studies are needed to determine the optimal preoperative evaluation of LVOT obstruction and potential treatments for LVOT obstruction associated with TMVR.

SUMMARY AND FUTURE DIRECTIONS

Patients with CKD and ESRD represent a population with high surgical risk and high prevalence of severe VHD. Outcomes of this population compared with patients without renal dysfunction are worse, and percutaneous procedures present an alternative with less risk compared with open cardiac surgery. AKI remains a significant perioperative complication that is predictive of poor outcomes; stringent protocols and a team-based approach are needed to avoid this complication. Given the expanding indications for percutaneous structural interventions, further research is needed to identify ideal patients with CKD or ESRD who would benefit from intervention.

CLINICS CARE POINTS

- Periprocedural AKI after structural intervention is associated with increased morbidity and mortality.

- Pre, during and post procedural hemodynamic optimization are critical for prevention of AKI. Minimization of hypotension, low cardiac output situations and contrast load can be beneficial. Optimization of hemodynamics and procedural outcomes should be the goal with low threshold for invasive monitoring in high risk patients.

- TAVR is associated with a lower risk of periprocedural AKI compared to SAVR, and may improve CKD stage by alleviating cardiorenal syndrome caused by AS.

- Patient selection is critical in determining which patients with CKD or ESRD will do well post-TAVR, but compared to SAVR, TAVR is still associated with lower morbidity and mortality in this population.

CONFLICTS OF INTEREST

The authors declare no conflicts of interest.

REFERENCES

1. Bach DS, Siao D, Girard SE, et al. Evaluation of patients with severe symptomatic aortic stenosis who do not undergo aortic valve replacement: the potential role of subjectively overestimated operative risk. Circ Cardiovasc Qual Outcomes 2009;2:533–9.
2. Pellikka PA, Sarano ME, Nishimura RA, et al. Outcome of 622 adults with asymptomatic, hemodynamically significant aortic stenosis during prolonged follow-up. Circulation 2005;111:3290–5.
3. Coisne A, Montaigne D, Aghezzaf S, et al. Association of mortality with aortic stenosis severity in outpatients: results from the VALVENOR Study. JAMA Cardiol 2021;6:1424–31.
4. Turina J, Hess O, Sepulcri F, et al. Spontaneous course of aortic valve disease. Eur Heart J 1987; 8:471–83.
5. Sundt TM, Jneid H. Guideline update on indications for transcatheter aortic valve implantation based on the 2020 American College of Cardiology/American Heart Association guidelines for management of valvular heart disease. JAMA Cardiol 2021;6:1088–9. Available at: http://www.ncbi. nlm.nih.gov/pubmed/34287627.
6. Baldus S, Schillinger W, Franzen O, et al. MitraClip therapy in daily clinical practice: initial results from the German transcatheter mitral valve interventions (TRAMI) registry. Eur J Heart Fail 2012;14: 1050–5.
7. Glower DD, Kar S, Trento A, et al. Percutaneous mitral valve repair for mitral regurgitation in high-risk patients: results of the EVEREST II study. J Am Coll Cardiol 2014;64:172–81.
8. Maisano F, Franzen O, Baldus S, et al. Percutaneous mitral valve interventions in the real world: early and 1-year results from the ACCESS-EU, a prospective, multicenter, nonrandomized post-approval study of the MitraClip therapy in Europe. J Am Coll Cardiol 2013;62:1052–61.
9. Nickenig G, Estevez-Loureiro R, Franzen O, et al. Percutaneous mitral valve edge-to-edge repair: in-hospital results and 1-year follow-up of 628 patients of the 2011-2012 pilot European Sentinel Registry. J Am Coll Cardiol 2014;64:875–84.
10. Kappetein AP, Head SJ, Généreux P, et al. Updated standardized endpoint definitions for transcatheter aortic valve implantation: the Valve Academic Research Consortium-2 consensus document (varc-2). Eur J Cardio-thoracic Surg 2012;42.
11. Mehta RL, Kellum JA, Shah SV, et al. Acute Kidney Injury Network: report of an initiative to improve outcomes in acute kidney injury. Crit Care 2007; 11:1–8.
12. Kellum JA, Lameire N, Aki K, et al. KDIGO AKI Guideline Work Group. Diagnosis, evaluation, and management of acute kidney injury: a KDIGO summary. Crit Care 2013;17:1–15. Available at: https://pubmed.ncbi.nlm.nih.gov/23394211/.
13. Généreux P, Piazza N, Alu MC, et al. Valve Academic Research Consortium 3: updated endpoint definitions for aortic valve clinical research. Eur Heart J 2021;42:1825–57.
14. Shacham Y, Rofe M, Leshem-Rubinow E, et al. Usefulness of urine output criteria for early detection of acute kidney injury after transcatheter aortic valve implantation. Cardiorenal Med 2014; 4:155–60.
15. Koifman E, Segev A, Fefer P, et al. Comparison of acute kidney injury classifications in patients undergoing transcatheter aortic valve implantation: predictors and long-term outcomes. Cathet Cardiovasc Interv 2016;87:523–31.
16. Saia F, Ciuca C, Taglieri N, et al. Acute kidney injury following transcatheter aortic valve implantation: incidence, predictors and clinical outcome. Int J Cardiol 2013;168:1034–40.
17. Wang J, Yu W, Zhou Y, et al. Independent risk factors contributing to acute kidney injury according to updated Valve Academic Research Consortium-2 criteria after transcatheter aortic valve implantation: a meta-analysis and meta-regression of 13 studies. J Cardiothorac Vasc Anesth 2017;31:816–26.
18. Bagur R, Webb JG, Nietlispach F, et al. Acute kidney injury following transcatheter aortic valve implantation: predictive factors, prognostic value, and comparison with surgical aortic valve replacement. Eur Heart J 2010;31:865–74.

19. Nuis RJM, Van Mieghem NM, Tzikas A, et al. Frequency, determinants, and prognostic effects of acute kidney injury and red blood cell transfusion in patients undergoing transcatheter aortic valve implantation. Cathet Cardiovasc Interv 2011;77: 881–9.

20. Alassar A, Roy D, Abdulkareem N, et al. Acute kidney injury after transcatheter aortic valve implantation: incidence, risk factors, and prognostic effects. Innovations 2012;7:389–93. Available at: http://www.ncbi.nlm.nih.gov/pubmed/23422799.

21. Abbas S, Qayum I, Wahid R, et al. Acute kidney injury in transcatheter aortic valve replacement. Cureus 2021;13:10–2.

22. Crowhurst JA, Savage M, Subban V, et al. Factors contributing to acute kidney injury and the impact on mortality in patients undergoing transcatheter aortic valve replacement. Hear Lung Circ 2016;25: 282–9.

23. Konigstein M, Ben-Assa E, Abramowitz Y, et al. Usefulness of updated Valve Academic Research Consortium-2 criteria for acute kidney injury following transcatheter aortic valve implantation. Am J Cardiol 2013;112:1807–11.

24. Oguri A, Yamamoto M, Mouillet G, et al. Impact of chronic kidney disease on the outcomes of transcatheter aortic valve implantation: results from the FRANCE 2 registry. EuroIntervention 2015;10:e1–9. Available at: http://www.ncbi.nlm. nih.gov/pubmed/25599700.

25. Sinning JM, Ghanem A, Steinhuser H, et al. Renal function as predictor of mortality in patients after percutaneous transcatheter aortic valve implantation. JACC Cardiovasc Interv 2010;3:1141–9.

26. Anand IS, Chandrashekhar Y, Ferrari R, et al. Pathogenesis of congestive state in chronic obstructive pulmonary disease. Studies of body water and sodium, renal function, hemodynamics, and plasma hormones during edema and after recovery. Circulation 1992;86:12–21. Available at: http://www.ncbi.nlm.nih.gov/pubmed/1617764.

27. Nso N, Emmanuel K, Nassar M, et al. Impact of new-onset versus pre-existing atrial fibrillation on outcomes after transcatheter aortic valve replacement/implantation. IJC Hear Vasc 2022;38:100910.

28. Schefold JC, Filippatos G, Hasenfuss G, et al. Heart failure and kidney dysfunction: epidemiology, mechanisms and management. Nat Rev Nephrol 2016;12:610–23.

29. Scherner M, Wahlers T. Acute kidney injury after transcatheter aortic valve implantation. J Thorac Dis 2015;7:1527–35.

30. Ozkok A. Cholesterol-embolization syndrome: current perspectives. Vasc Health Risk Manag 2019;15: 209–20. Available at: https://www.dovepress.com/ cholesterol-embolization-syndrome-current-per-spectives-peer-reviewed-article-VHRM.

31. Ram P, Mezue K, Pressman G, et al. Acute kidney injury post–transcatheter aortic valve replacement. Clin Cardiol 2017;40:1357–62.

32. Thongprayoon C, Cheungpasitporn W, Srivali N, et al. Acute kidney injury after transcatheter aortic valve replacement: a systematic review and meta-analysis. Am J Nephrol 2015;41:372–82. Available at: http://www.ncbi.nlm.nih.gov/pubmed/26113391.

33. Van Mieghem NM, Schipper MEI, Ladich E, et al. Histopathology of embolic debris captured during transcatheter aortic valve replacement. Circulation 2013;127:2194–201.

34. Kapadia SR, Kodali S, Makkar R, et al. Protection against cerebral embolism during transcatheter aortic valve replacement. J Am Coll Cardiol 2017;69:367–77.

35. Ranasinghe MP, Peter K, McFadyen JD. Thromboembolic and bleeding complications in transcatheter aortic valve implantation: insights on mechanisms, prophylaxis and therapy. J Clin Med 2019;8:1–16.

36. Shishikura D, Kataoka Y, Pisaniello AD, et al. The extent of aortic atherosclerosis predicts the occurrence, severity, and recovery of acute kidney injury after transcatheter aortic valve replacement: a volumetric multislice computed tomography analysis. Circ Cardiovasc Interv 2018;11:1–11.

37. Alzu'bi H, Rmilah AA, Haq I-U, et al. Effect of TAVR approach and other baseline factors on the incidence of acute kidney injury: a systematic review and meta-analysis. J Intervent Cardiol 2022;2022:1–9.

38. Nuis RJ, Rodés-Cabau J, Sinning JM, et al. Blood transfusion and the risk of acute kidney injury after transcatheter aortic valve implantation. Circ Cardiovasc Interv 2012;5:680–8.

39. Aregger F, Wenaweser P, Hellige GJ, et al. Risk of acute kidney injury in patients with severe aortic valve stenosis undergoing transcatheter valve replacement. Nephrol Dial Transplant 2009;24: 2175–9.

40. Malhotra G, Chua S, Kodumuri V, et al. Rare presentation of lupus myocarditis with acute heart failure: a case report. Am J Therapeut 2016;23: e1952–5. Available at: http://www.lww.com/ store/products?1075-2765%0Ahttp://ovidsp.ovid. com/ovidweb.cgi?T=JS&CSC=Y&NEWS=N& PAGE=fulltext&D=emed18b&AN=606981459.

41. Seeger J, Kapadia SR, Kodali S, et al. Rate of periprocedural stroke observed with cerebral embolic protection during transcatheter aortic valve replacement: a patient-level propensity-matched analysis. Eur Heart J 2019;40:1334–9.

42. Barbash IM, Ben-Dor I, Dvir D, et al. Incidence and predictors of acute kidney injury after transcatheter aortic valve replacement. Am Heart J 2012; 163:1031–6.

43. Kong WY, Yong G, Irish A. Incidence, risk factors and prognosis of acute kidney injury after transcatheter aortic valve implantation. Nephrology 2012;17:445–51.

44. Kumar N, Khera R, Fonarow GC, et al. Comparison of outcomes of transfemoral versus transapical approach for transcatheter aortic valve implantation. Am J Cardiol 2018;122:1520–6.

45. Ribeiro HB, Dahou A, Urena M, et al. Myocardial injury after transaortic versus transapical transcatheter aortic valve replacement. Ann Thorac Surg 2015;99:2001–9.

46. Najjar M, Salna M, George I. Acute kidney injury after aortic valve replacement: incidence, risk factors and outcomes. Expert Rev Cardiovasc Ther 2015;13:301–16.

47. Kliuk-Ben Bassat O, Finkelstein A, Bazan S, et al. Acute kidney injury after transcatheter aortic valve implantation and mortality risk: long-term follow-up. Nephrol Dial Transplant 2020;35:433–8.

48. Wystub N, Bäz L, Möbius-Winkler S, et al. Aortic annulus measurement with computed tomography angiography reduces aortic regurgitation after transfemoral aortic valve replacement compared to 3-D echocardiography: a single-centre experience. Clin Res Cardiol 2019;108:1266–75.

49. Asami M, Pilgrim T, Stortecky S, et al. Impact of valvular resistance on aortic regurgitation after transcatheter aortic valve replacement according to the type of prosthesis. Clin Res Cardiol 2019;108:1343–53.

50. Mauri V, Körber MI, Kuhn E, et al. Prognosis of persistent mitral regurgitation in patients undergoing transcatheter aortic valve replacement. Clin Res Cardiol 2020;109:1261–70.

51. Wernly B, Seelmaier C, Leistner D, et al. Mechanical circulatory support with Impella versus intra-aortic balloon pump or medical treatment in cardiogenic shock: a critical appraisal of current data. Clin Res Cardiol 2019;108:1249–57.

52. Wernly B, Eder S, Navarese EP, et al. Transcatheter aortic valve replacement for pure aortic valve regurgitation: "on-label" versus "off-label" use of TAVR devices. Clin Res Cardiol 2019;108:921–30.

53. Wernly B, Zappe AK, Unbehaun A, et al. Transcatheter valve-in-valve implantation (VinV-TAVR) for failed surgical aortic bioprosthetic valves. Clin Res Cardiol 2019;108:83–92.

54. Thiele RH, Isbell JM, Rosner MH. AKI associated with cardiac surgery. Clin J Am Soc Nephrol 2015;10:500–14. Available at: http://www.ncbi.nlm.nih.gov/pubmed/25376763.

55. McIlroy DR, Lopez MG, Billings FT. Perioperative clinical trials in AKI. Semin Nephrol 2020;40:173–87.

56. Malek M, Nematbakhsh M. Renal ischemia/reperfusion injury; from pathophysiology to treatment. J Ren Inj Prev 2015;4:20–7. Available at: http://www.ncbi.nlm.nih.gov/pubmed/26060833%0Ahttp://www.pubmedcentral.nih.gov/articlerender.fcgi?artid=PMC4459724.

57. Bove T, Calabrò MG, Landoni G, et al. The incidence and risk of acute renal failure after cardiac surgery. J Cardiothorac Vasc Anesth 2004;18:442–5.

58. Grayson AD, Khater M, Jackson M, et al. Valvular heart operation is an independent risk factor for acute renal failure. Ann Thorac Surg 2003;75:1829–35.

59. Karkouti K, Wijeysundera DN, Yau TM, et al. Acute kidney injury after cardiac surgery. Focus on modifiable risk factors. Circulation 2009;119:495–502.

60. Murashita T, Greason KL, Suri RM, et al. Aortic valve replacement for severe aortic valve stenosis in the nonagenarian patient. Ann Thorac Surg 2014;98:1593–7.

61. Mehran R, Dangas GD, Weisbord SD. Contrast-associated acute kidney injury. N Engl J Med 2019;380:2146–55.

62. McDonald JS, Leake CB, McDonald RJ, et al. Acute kidney injury after intravenous versus intra-arterial contrast material administration in a paired cohort. Invest Radiol 2016;51:804–9.

63. McDonald JS, McDonald RJ, Carter RE, et al. Risk of intravenous contrast material-mediated acute kidney injury: a propensity score-matched study stratified by baseline-estimated glomerular filtration rate. Radiology 2014;271:65–73.

64. McDonald RJ, McDonald JS, Carter RE, et al. Intravenous contrast material exposure is not an independent risk factor for dialysis or mortality. Radiology 2014;273:714–25.

65. McDonald RJ, McDonald JS, Bida JP, et al. Intravenous contrast material-induced nephropathy: causal or coincident phenomenon? Radiology 2013;267:106–18.

66. Miura D, Yamada Y, Kusaba S, et al. Influence of preoperative serum creatinine level and intraoperative volume of contrast medium on the risk of acute kidney injury after transfemoral transcatheter aortic valve implantation: a retrospective observational study. BMC Res Notes 2019;12:1–6.

67. Gul I, Zungur M, Tastan A, et al. The importance of contrast volume/glomerular filtration rate ratio in contrast-induced nephropathy patients after transcatheter aortic valve implantation. Cardiorenal Med 2015;5:31–9.

68. Su X, Xie X, Liu L, et al. Comparative effectiveness of 12 treatment strategies for preventing contrast-induced acute kidney injury: a systematic review and Bayesian network meta-analysis. Am J Kidney Dis 2017;69:69–77.

69. Kelly AM, Dwamena B, Cronin P, et al. Review Annals of Internal Medicine meta-analysis: effectiveness of drugs for preventing contrast-induced nephropathy. Ann Intern Med 2014;148:1434–45.

70. Leon MB, Smith CR, Mack M, et al. Transcatheter aortic-valve implantation for aortic stenosis in patients who cannot undergo surgery. N Engl J Med 2010;363:1597–607. Available at: http://www.ncbi.nlm.nih.gov/pubmed/20961243.

71. Leon MB, Smith CR, Mack MJ, et al. Transcatheter or surgical aortic-valve replacement in intermediate-risk patients. N Engl J Med 2016;374:1609–20.

72. Smith CR, Leon MB, Mack MJ, et al. Transcatheter versus surgical aortic-valve replacement in high-risk patients. N Engl J Med 2011;364:2187–98. Available at: http://www.ncbi.nlm.nih.gov/pubmed/21639811.

73. Mack MJ, Leon MB, Thourani VH, et al. Transcatheter aortic-valve replacement with a balloon-expandable valve in low-risk patients. N Engl J Med 2019;380:1695–705.

74. Thongprayoon C, Cheungpasitporn W, Srivali N, et al. AKI after transcatheter or surgical aortic valve replacement. J Am Soc Nephrol 2016;27:1854–60. Available at: http://www.ncbi.nlm.nih.gov/pubmed/26487562.

75. Arbel Y, Ben-Assa E, Puzhevsky D, et al. Forced diuresis with matched hydration during transcatheter aortic valve implantation for Reducing Acute Kidney Injury: A randomized, sham-controlled study (REDUCE-AKI). Eur Heart J 2019;40:3169–78.

76. Attard S, Buttigieg J, Galea S, et al. The incidence, predictors, and prognosis of acute kidney injury after transcatheter aortic valve implantation. Clin Nephrol 2018;90:373–9. Available at: http://www.ncbi.nlm.nih.gov/pubmed/30369403.

77. Strauch JT, Scherner MP, Haldenwang PL, et al. Minimally invasive transapical aortic valve implantation and the risk of acute kidney injury. Ann Thorac Surg 2010;89:465–70.

78. Adams DH, Popma JJ, Reardon MJ, et al. Transcatheter aortic-valve replacement with a self-expanding prosthesis. N Engl J Med 2014;370:1790–8.

79. Reardon MJ, Van Mieghem NM, Popma JJ, et al. Surgical or transcatheter aortic-valve replacement in intermediate-risk patients. N Engl J Med 2017;376:1321–31.

80. Popma JJ, Deeb GM, Yakubov SJ, et al. Transcatheter aortic-valve replacement with a self-expanding valve in low-risk patients. N Engl J Med 2019;380:1706–15.

81. Barbanti M, Gulino S, Capranzano P, et al. Acute kidney injury with the RenalGuard system in patients undergoing transcatheter aortic valve replacement: the PROTECT-TAVI Trial (PROphylactic effecT of furosEmide-induCed diuresis with matched isotonic intravenous hydraTion in Transcatheter Aortic Va. JACC Cardiovasc Interv 2015;8:1595–604.

82. Villablanca PA, Mathew V, Thourani VH, et al. A meta-analysis and meta-regression of long-term outcomes of transcatheter versus surgical aortic valve replacement for severe aortic stenosis. Int J Cardiol 2016;225:234–43.

83. Durand E, Avinée G, Gillibert A, et al. Analysis of length of stay after transfemoral transcatheter aortic valve replacement: results from the FRANCE TAVI registry. Clin Res Cardiol 2021;110:40–9.

84. Witberg G, Steinmetz T, Landes U, et al. Change in kidney function and 2-year mortality after transcatheter aortic valve replacement. JAMA Netw Open 2021;4:1–13.

85. Fu J, Popal MS, Li Y, et al. Transcatheter versus surgical aortic valve replacement in low and intermediate risk patients with severe aortic stenosis: systematic review and meta-analysis of randomized controlled trials and propensity score matching observational studies. J Thorac Dis 2019;11:1945–62.

86. Latif A, Ahsan MJ, Lateef N, et al. Outcomes of surgical versus transcatheter aortic valve replacement in nonagenarians: a systematic review and meta-analysis. J Community Hosp Intern Med Perspect 2021;11:128–34.

87. Lou Y, Gao Y, Yu Y, et al. Efficacy and safety of transcatheter vs. surgical aortic valve replacement in low-to-intermediate-risk patients: a meta-analysis. Front Cardiovasc Med 2020;7.

88. Shah K, Chaker Z, Busu T, et al. Meta-analysis comparing renal outcomes after transcatheter versus surgical aortic valve replacement. J Intervent Cardiol 2019;2019.

89. Feldman T, Foster E, Glower DD, et al. Percutaneous repair or surgery for mitral regurgitation. N Engl J Med 2011;364:1395–406. Available at: http://www.ncbi.nlm.nih.gov/pubmed/21463154.

90. Stone GW, Lindenfeld J, Abraham WT, et al. Transcatheter mitral-valve repair in patients with heart failure. N Engl J Med 2018;379:2307–18.

91. Obadia J-F, Messika-Zeitoun D, Leurent G, et al. Percutaneous repair or medical treatment for secondary mitral regurgitation. N Engl J Med 2018;379:2297–306.

92. Armijo G, Estevez-Loureiro R, Carrasco-Chinchilla F, et al. Acute kidney injury after percutaneous edge-to-edge mitral repair. J Am Coll Cardiol 2020;76:2463–73.

93. Tonchev I, Heberman D, Peretz A, et al. Acute kidney injury after MitraClip implantation in patients with severe mitral regurgitation. Cathet Cardiovasc Interv 2021;97:E868–74.

94. Doulamis IP, Tzani A, Kampaktsis PN, et al. Acute kidney injury following transcatheter edge-to-

edge mitral valve repair: a systematic review and meta-analysis. Cardiovasc Revascularization Med 2022;38:29–35.

95. Spieker M, Hellhammer K, Katsianos S, et al. Effect of acute kidney injury after percutaneous mitral valve repair on outcome. Am J Cardiol 2018;122:316–22.

96. Nazir S, Ahuja KR, Kolte D, et al. Association of acute kidney injury with outcomes in patients undergoing transcatheter mitral valve repair. Cardiol 2021;146:501–7.

97. Chandrashekhar Y, Westaby S, Narula J. Mitral stenosis. Lancet 2009;374:1271–83.

98. Badheka AO, Shah N, Ghatak A, et al. Balloon mitral valvuloplasty in the United States: a 13-year perspective. Am J Med 2014;127:1126.e1–12.

99. Nkomo VT, Gardin JM, Skelton TN, et al. Burden of valvular heart diseases: a population-based study. Lancet 2006;368:1005–11.

100. Palacios IF. Percutaneous mitral balloon valvuloplasty: worldwide trends. J Am Heart Assoc 2019;8:1–3.

101. Slehria T, Hendrickson MJ, Sivaraj K, et al. Trends in percutaneous balloon mitral valvuloplasty complications for mitral stenosis in the United States (the National Inpatient Sample [2008 to 2018]). Am J Cardiol 2022;182:77–82.

102. Samad Z, Sivak JA, Phelan M, et al. Prevalence and outcomes of left-sided valvular heart disease associated with chronic kidney disease. J Am Heart Assoc 2017;6:1–14.

103. Rodés-Cabau J, Webb JG, Cheung A, et al. Transcatheter aortic valve implantation for the treatment of severe symptomatic aortic stenosis in patients at very high or prohibitive surgical risk. Acute and late outcomes of the multicenter Canadian experience. J Am Coll Cardiol 2010;55:1080–90.

104. Wessely M, Rau S, Lange P, et al. Chronic kidney disease is not associated with a higher risk for mortality or acute kidney injury in transcatheter aortic valve implantation. Nephrol Dial Transplant 2012;27:3502–8.

105. Ix JH, Shlipak MG, Katz R, et al. Kidney function and aortic valve and mitral annular calcification in the Multi-Ethnic Study of Atherosclerosis (MESA). Am J Kidney Dis 2007;50:412–20.

106. Rattazzi M, Bertacco E, Del Vecchio A, et al. Aortic valve calcification in chronic kidney disease. Nephrol Dial Transplant 2013;28:2968–76.

107. Levin NW, Hoenich NA. Consequences of hyperphosphatemia and elevated levels of the calcium-phosphorus product in dialysis patients. Curr Opin Nephrol Hypertens 2001;10:563–8.

108. Merjanian R, Budoff M, Adler S, et al. Coronary artery, aortic wall, and valvular calcification in nondialyzed individuals with type 2 diabetes and renal disease. Kidney Int 2003;64:263–71.

109. Saran R, Robinson B, Abbott KC, et al. US Renal Data System 2017 Annual Data Report: epidemiology of kidney disease in the United States. Am J Kidney Dis 2018;71:A7.

110. Cianciolo G, Capelli I, Angelini ML, et al. Importance of vascular calcification in kidney transplant recipients. Am J Nephrol 2014;39:418–26.

111. Perkovic V, Hunt D, Griffin SV, et al. Accelerated progression of calcific aortic stenosis in dialysis patients. Nephron Clin Pract 2004;94:c40–5. Available at: https://www.karger.com/Article/FullText/71280.

112. O'Neill WC, Lomashvili KA. Recent progress in the treatment of vascular calcification. Kidney Int 2010;78:1232–9. Available at: http://www.ncbi.nlm.nih.gov/pubmed/20861819.

113. Maher ER, Young G, Smyth-Walsh B, et al. Aortic and mitral valve calcification in patients with end-stage renal disease. Lancet 1987;330:875–7.

114. Wang AYM, Woo J, Wang M, et al. Association of inflammation and malnutrition with cardiac valve calcification in continuous ambulatory peritoneal dialysis patients. J Am Soc Nephrol 2001;12:1927–36. Available at: http://www.ncbi.nlm.nih.gov/pubmed/11518787.

115. Yutzey KE, Demer LL, Body SC, et al. Calcific aortic valve disease: a consensus summary from the alliance of investigators on calcific aortic valve disease. Arterioscler Thromb Vasc Biol 2014;34:2387–93.

116. Schlieper G, Schurgers L, Brandenburg V, et al. Vascular calcification in chronic kidney disease: an update. Nephrol Dial Transplant 2016;31:31–9.

117. Brandenburg VM, Schuh A, Kramann R. Valvular calcification in chronic kidney disease. Adv Chron Kidney Dis 2019;26:464–71.

118. Cianciolo G, Galassi A, Capelli I, et al. Klotho-FGF23, cardiovascular disease, and vascular calcification: black or white? Curr Vasc Pharmacol 2018;16:143–56. Available at: http://www.ncbi.nlm.nih.gov/pubmed/28294047.

119. Price PA, Faus SA, Williamson MK. Warfarin causes rapid calcification of the elastic lamellae in rat arteries and heart valves. Arterioscler Thromb Vasc Biol 1998;18:1400–7.

120. Alappan HR, Kaur G, Manzoor S, et al. Warfarin accelerates medial arterial calcification in humans. Arterioscler Thromb Vasc Biol 2020;1413–9.

121. de Vriese AS, Caluwé R, Pyfferoen L, et al. Multicenter randomized controlled trial of vitamin K antagonist replacement by rivaroxaban with or without vitamin K2 in hemodialysis patients with atrial fibrillation: the Valkyrie study. J Am Soc Nephrol 2020;31:186–96.

122. Alkhouli M, Alasfar S, Samuels LA. Valvular heart disease and dialysis access: a case of cardiac decompensation after fistula creation. J Vasc Access 2013;14:96. Available at: http://www.ncbi.nlm.nih.gov/pubmed/22865537.

123. Cirit M, Özkahya M, Çinar CS, et al. Disappearance of mitral and tricuspid regurgitation in haemodialysis patients after ultrafiltration. Nephrol Dial Transplant 1998;13:389–92.

124. Massera D, Trivieri MG, Andrews JPM, et al. Disease activity in mitral annular calcification: a multimodality study. Circ Cardiovasc Imaging 2019;12:1–10.

125. Abramowitz Y, Jilaihawi H, Chakravarty T, et al. Mitral annulus calcification. J Am Coll Cardiol 2015;66:1934–41.

126. Abd alamir M, Radulescu V, Goyfman M, et al. Prevalence and correlates of mitral annular calcification in adults with chronic kidney disease: results from CRIC study. Atherosclerosis 2015;242:117–22.

127. Ward C. Clinical significance of the bicuspid aortic valve. Heart 2000;83:81–5.

128. Umana E, Ahmed W, Alpert MA. Valvular and perivalvular abnormalities in end-stage renal disease. Am J Med Sci 2003;325:237–42. Available at: http://www.ncbi.nlm.nih.gov/pubmed/12695729.

129. Dvir D, Bourguignon T, Otto CM, et al. Standardized definition of structural valve degeneration for surgical and transcatheter bioprosthetic aortic valves. Circulation 2018;137:388–99.

130. Ennezat PV, Maréchaux S, Pibarot P. From excessive high-flow, high-gradient to paradoxical low-flow, low-gradient aortic valve stenosis: hemodialysis arteriovenous fistula model. Cardiology 2010;116:70–2.

131. Bradley SM, Foag K, Monteagudo K, et al. Use of routinely captured echocardiographic data in the diagnosis of severe aortic stenosis. Heart 2019;105:112–6.

132. Finegold JA, Manisty CH, Cecaro F, et al. Choosing between velocity-time-integral ratio and peak velocity ratio for calculation of the dimensionless index (or aortic valve area) in serial follow-up of aortic stenosis. Int J Cardiol 2013;167:1524–31.

133. Rusinaru D, Malaquin D, Maréchaux S, et al. Relation of dimensionless index to long-term outcome in aortic stenosis with preserved LVEF. JACC Cardiovasc Imaging 2015;8:766–75.

134. Clavel MA, Messika-Zeitoun D, Pibarot P, et al. The complex nature of discordant severe calcified aortic valve disease grading: new insights from combined Doppler echocardiographic and computed tomographic study. J Am Coll Cardiol 2013;62:2329–38.

135. Cavallo AU, Patterson AJ, Thomas R, et al. Low dose contrast CT for transcatheter aortic valve replacement assessment: results from the prospective SPECTACULAR study (spectral CT assessment prior to TAVR). J Cardiovasc Comput Tomogr 2020;14:68–74.

136. Hana D, Miller T, Skaff P, et al. 3D transesophageal echocardiography for guiding transcatheter aortic valve replacement without prior cardiac computed tomography in patients with renal dysfunction. Cardiovasc Revascularization Med 2022;41:63–8.

137. Wang J, Jagasia DH, Kondapally YR, et al. Comparison of non-contrast cardiovascular magnetic resonance imaging to computed tomography angiography for aortic annular sizing before transcatheter aortic valve replacement. J Invasive Cardiol 2017;29:239–45. Available at: http://www.ncbi.nlm.nih.gov/pubmed/28570260.

138. Weinreb JC, Rodby RA, Yee J, et al. Use of intravenous gadolinium-based contrast media in patients with kidney disease: consensus statements from the American College of Radiology and the National Kidney Foundation. Radiology 2021;298:28–35.

139. Francone M, Budde RPJ, Bremerich J, et al. CT and MR imaging prior to transcatheter aortic valve implantation: standardisation of scanning protocols, measurements and reporting—a consensus document by the European Society of Cardiovascular Radiology (ESCR). Eur Radiol 2020;30:2627–50. Available at: http://link.springer.com/10.1007/s00330-019-06357-8.

140. Carabello BA. The SEAS trial. Curr Cardiol Rep 2010;12:122–4.

141. O'Brien KD, Probstfield JL, Caulfield MT, et al. Angiotensin-converting enzyme inhibitors and change in aortic valve calcium. Arch Intern Med 2005;165:858–62.

142. Rosenhek R, Rader F, Loho N, et al. Statins but not angiotensin-converting enzyme inhibitors delay progression of aortic stenosis. Circulation 2004;110:1291–5.

143. Raggi P, Chertow GM, Torres PU, et al. The ADVANCE study: a randomized study to evaluate the effects of cinacalcet plus low-dose vitamin D on vascular calcification in patients on hemodialysis. Nephrol Dial Transplant 2011;26:1327–39.

144. The EVOLVE Trial Investigators. Effect of cinacalcet on cardiovascular disease in patients undergoing dialysis. N Engl J Med 2012;367:2482–94. Available at: http://www.nejm.org/doi/abs/10.1056/NEJMoa1205624.

145. Pawade TA, Doris MK, Bing R, et al. Effect of denosumab or alendronic acid on the progression of aortic stenosis: a double-blind randomized controlled trial. Circulation 2021;143:2418–27.

146. Straumann E, Meyer B, Misteli M, et al. Aortic and mitral valve disease in patients with end stage renal failure on long-term haemodialysis. Br Heart J 1992;67:236–9.

147. Thourani VH, Sarin EL, Keeling WB, et al. Long-term survival for patients with preoperative renal failure undergoing bioprosthetic or mechanical valve replacement. Ann Thorac Surg 2011;91:1127–34.

148. Horst M, Mehlhorn U, Hoerstrup SP, et al. Cardiac surgery in patients with end-stage renal disease: 10-year experience. Ann Thorac Surg 2000;69: 96–101. Available at: https://linkinghub.elsevier.com/retrieve/pii/S0003497599011339.

149. Brennan JM, Edwards FH, Zhao Y, et al. Long-term survival after aortic valve replacement among high-risk elderly patients in the United States: insights from the Society of Thoracic Surgeons adult cardiac surgery database, 1991 to 2007. Circulation 2012;126:1621–9.

150. Garcia S, Cubeddu RJ, Hahn RT, et al. 5-Year outcomes comparing surgical versus transcatheter aortic valve replacement in patients with chronic kidney disease. JACC Cardiovasc Interv 2021;14: 1995–2005.

151. Cubeddu RJ, Asher CR, Lowry AM, et al. Impact of transcatheter aortic valve replacement on severity of chronic kidney disease. J Am Coll Cardiol 2020; 76:1410–21.

152. Wang J, Liu S, Han X, et al. Impact of chronic kidney disease on the prognosis of transcatheter aortic valve replacement in patients with aortic stenosis: a meta-analysis of 133624 patients. Ann Thorac Cardiovasc Surg 2022;28:83–95.

153. Szerlip M, Zajarias A, Vemalapalli S, et al. Transcatheter aortic valve replacement in patients with end-stage renal disease. J Am Coll Cardiol 2019;73:2806–15.

154. Allende R, Webb JG, Munoz-Garcia AJ, et al. Advanced chronic kidney disease in patients undergoing transcatheter aortic valve implantation: insights on clinical outcomes and prognostic markers from a large cohort of patients. Eur Heart J 2014;35:2685–96.

155. Thourani VH, Forcillo J, Beohar N, et al. Impact of preoperative chronic kidney disease in 2,531 high-risk and inoperable patients undergoing transcatheter aortic valve replacement in the PARTNER trial. Ann Thorac Surg 2016;102: 1172–80.

156. Szerlip M, Kim RJ, Adeniyi T, et al. The outcomes of transcatheter aortic valve replacement in a cohort of patients with end-stage renal disease. Cathet Cardiovasc Interv 2016;87:1314–21.

157. Hansen JW, Foy A, Yadav P, et al. Death and dialysis after transcatheter aortic valve replacement: an analysis of the STS/ACC TVT Registry. JACC Cardiovasc Interv 2017;10:2064–75.

158. Gupta T, Goel K, Kolte D, et al. Association of chronic kidney disease with in-hospital outcomes of transcatheter aortic valve replacement. JACC Cardiovasc Interv 2017;10:2050–60.

159. Puri R, Iung B, Cohen DJ, et al. TAVI or no TAVI: identifying patients unlikely to benefit from transcatheter aortic valve implantation. Eur Heart J 2016;37:2217–25.

160. Urzua J, Troncoso S, Bugedo G, et al. Renal function and cardiopulmonary bypass: effect of perfusion pressure. J Cardiothorac Vasc Anesth 1992;6: 299–303.

161. Ling LG, Zeng N, Liu J, et al. Risk factors for acute kidney injury following 5100 cardiac surgeries with extracorporeal circulation. Zhong Nan Da Xue Bugged Bao Yi Xue Ban 2009;34:861–6. Available at: http://www.ncbi.nlm.nih.gov/pubmed/19779257.

162. Sreeram GM, Grocott HP, White WD, et al. Transcranial Doppler emboli count predicts rise in creatinine after coronary artery bypass graft surgery. J Cardiothorac Vasc Anesth 2004;18:548–51.

163. Cheng X, Hu Q, Zhao H, et al. Transcatheter versus surgical aortic valve replacement in patients with chronic kidney disease: a meta-analysis. J Cardiothorac Vasc Anesth 2019;33:2221–30.

164. Wei S, Zhang P, Zhai K, et al. Transcatheter versus surgical aortic valve replacement in aortic stenosis patients with advanced chronic kidney disease: a systematic review and meta-analysis. Ann Palliat Med 2021;10:7157–72.

165. Kaneko H, Neuss M, Schau T, et al. Interaction between renal function and percutaneous edge-to-edge mitral valve repair using MitraClip. J Cardiol 2017;69:476–82.

166. Vassileva CM, Brennan JM, Gammie JS, et al. Mitral procedure selection in patients on dialysis: does mitral repair influence outcomes? J Thorac Cardiovasc Surg 2014;148:144–50.e1.

167. Wang A, Sangli C, Lim S, et al. Evaluation of renal function before and after percutaneous mitral valve repair. Circ Cardiovasc Interv 2015;8:1–8.

168. Schueler R, Nickenig G, May AE, et al. Predictors for short-term outcomes of patients undergoing transcatheter mitral valve interventions: analysis of 778 prospective patients from the German TRAMI registry focusing on baseline renal function. EuroIntervention 2016;12:508–14. Available at: http://www.ncbi.nlm.nih.gov/pubmed/26348678.

169. Rassaf T, Balzer J, Rammos C, et al. Influence of percutaneous mitral valve repair using the MitraClip® system on renal function in patients with severe mitral regurgitation. Cathet Cardiovasc Interv 2015;85:899–903.

170. Kalbacher D, Daubmann A, Tigges E, et al. Impact of pre- and post-procedural renal dysfunction on long-term outcomes in patients undergoing MitraClip implantation: a retrospective analysis

from two German high-volume centres. Int J Cardiol 2020;300:87–92. Available at: http://www.ncbi.nlm.nih.gov/pubmed/31748183.

171. Estévez-Loureiro R, Settergren M, Pighi M, et al. Effect of advanced chronic kidney disease in clinical and echocardiographic outcomes of patients treated with MitraClip system. Int J Cardiol 2015; 198:75–80.

172. Yoon SH, Bleiziffer S, Latib A, et al. Predictors of left ventricular outflow tract obstruction after transcatheter mitral valve replacement. JACC Cardiovasc Interv 2019;12:182–93.

173. Guerrero M, Urena M, Himbert D, et al. 1-Year outcomes of transcatheter mitral valve replacement in patients with severe mitral annular calcification. J Am Coll Cardiol 2018;71:1841–53.

Acute Kidney Injury Management Strategies Peri-Cardiovascular Interventions

Sanjay Chaudhary, MBBS, MD[a],
Kianoush B. Kashani, MD, MSc, MS[b,c],*

KEYWORDS

- Acute kidney injury • Contrast media • Atheroembolism • Cardiorenal syndrome
- Cardiac intervention

KEY POINTS

- Acute kidney injury (AKI) is common in the peri-interventional period and is associated with significantly higher mortality and morbidity.
- Contrast exposure, hemodynamic changes, atheroembolism, use of concomitant nephrotoxins, and cardiorenal syndrome are among AKI's most common pathophysiology mechanisms following cardiac interventions.
- AKI in peri-interventional time is at least partially preventable.
- Limiting contrast dose and optimizing effective blood volume and other AKI risk factors can decrease AKI incidence after exposure to contrast media.

INTRODUCTION

Acute kidney injury (AKI) incidence following cardiac interventional studies is reported within 10% to 17%.[1–3] The AKI occurrence leads to prolonged hospital stays, higher readmission rates, and higher total health care costs.[4] In addition, data reveal higher inpatient mortalities, bleeding, and myocardial infarction rates regardless of the procedure type, for example, coronary,[5] peripheral arterial,[6,7] or transcatheter aortic valve replacement (TAVR) procedures.[8] Indeed, AKI is considered a mainstream quality metric for in-hospital cardiovascular disease procedures in the United States. The AKI events are tracked and reported in the context of the American College of Cardiology (ACC) and National Cardiovascular Data Registries (NCDR) for percutaneous coronary intervention (PCI), TAVR, and other percutaneous valvular interventions.

Although AKI has dire consequences, it is considered a preventable syndrome. In a recent randomized controlled trial (RCT), implementing a clinical decision support system resulted in significantly less risk of AKI following cardiac interventions.[9] Therefore, understanding its pathophysiology and implementing adequate and timely preventive measures could improve clinical outcomes among those requiring cardiac interventions.

There are several mechanisms suggested as underlying causes of AKI following cardiac interventions. Exposure to intra-arterial contrast media is one of the most commonly proposed underlying pathophysiologic mechanisms. Besides contrast-associated acute kidney injury (CA-AKI), other

[a] Department of Critical Care Medicine, Mayo Clinic, 4500 San Pablo Road South, Jacksonville, FL 32224, USA;
[b] Division of Nephrology and Hypertension, Department of Medicine, Mayo Clinic, 200 First Street Southwest, Rochester, MN 55905, USA; [c] Division of Pulmonary and Critical Care Medicine, Department of Medicine, Mayo Clinic, 200 First Street Southwest, Rochester, MN 55905, USA
* Corresponding author. Division of Nephrology and Hypertension, Mayo Clinic, 200 First Street Southwest, Rochester, MN 55905.
E-mail address: Kashani.Kianoush@mayo.edu

Intervent Cardiol Clin 12 (2023) 555–572
https://doi.org/10.1016/j.iccl.2023.06.008
2211-7458/23/© 2023 Elsevier Inc. All rights reserved.

factors implicated in the pathogenesis include hypotension, cardiogenic shock, atheroembolism, effective blood volume inadequacies, for example, hypovolemia or hypervolemia, and exposure to other nephrotoxic medications.

In this review, the authors describe the AKI-proposed pathophysiology mechanisms, its diagnosis, and management strategies when it occurs after cardiovascular interventions.

PATHOPHYSIOLOGY
Contrast-Associated Acute Kidney Injury

The terminology used to describe AKI following cardiovascular procedures involving contrast media administration has been revised over time as the understanding of mechanisms has evolved. Similarly, the criteria to define AKI associated with contrast use has changed along with definitions of AKI in other settings.[10,11] The terminology and definition of CA-AKI (Table 1) have been discussed in detail in Lalith Vemireddy and Shweta Bansal's article, "Contrast-Associated Acute Kidney Injury: Definitions, Epidemiology, Pathophysiology and Implications," in this issue.

Three proposed mechanisms for a decline in kidney function have been reported after contrast media exposure. These include the following: (1) glomerular hemodynamic changes; (2) contrast cytotoxicity: contrast media can activate free radicals and reactive oxygen species, which can cause tubular cell damage; and finally, (3) high osmolar load.[12,13] Lalith Vemireddy and Shweta Bansal's article, "Contrast-Associated Acute Kidney Injury: Definitions, Epidemiology, Pathophysiology and Implications," in this issue details of these mechanisms.

Risk factors for contrast-associated–acute kidney injury

The risk factors of AKI following exposure to contrast media could be divided into 2 categories, that is, patient and contrast media-related (Table 2). Chronic kidney disease (CKD) is the most influential risk factor among patient-related risk factors.[14–18] Among modifiable risk factors are low effective blood volume, concomitant use of nephrotoxins, contrast dose and type (high-osmolar and ionic contrast media), and repeated exposure to contrast media.[15,16,19–25] Also, there has been reports that the risk of AKI following intraarterial contrast media is more than intravenous (IV), which could be due to several factors, including increased kidney exposure, more invasive nature of procedures with intraarterial administration that can increase the risk of other events like atheroembolic events.

Although a small RCT has strengthened this argument,[26] several studies reported the incidence of AKI was the same after consecutive exposure to intraarterial and IV contrast media.[27–30]

Several predictive models are proposed to determine the overall risks of AKI following exposure to contrast media (see Emily A. Eitzman and colleagues' article, "Predicting Contrast-Induced Renal Complications," in this issue).[31,32] It is worth mentioning that the ability of these models to predict AKI is the same regardless of the contrast media exposures.[33,34]

ATHEROEMBOLISM

Atheroembolic renal disease (AERD), also known as cholesterol atheroembolic renal disease, atheroembolism, cholesterol embolism, or cholesterol crystal embolization, is often regarded as an underdiagnosed clinical illness.[35,36] AERD is often considered an iatrogenic disease, as destabilizing atherosclerotic plaques during vascular manipulations could increase its risk substantially. AERD may follow surgical procedures like coronary artery bypass grafting, abdominal aortic aneurysm repair, and vascular procedures like angiography, angioplasty, or endovascular grafting. Simultaneous use of anticoagulants, that is, warfarin, heparin, antiplatelet agents, or thrombolytic therapies, increases the risk of AERD. AERD may occur spontaneously without inciting or triggering factors in a small proportion of patients.[37–39]

Although AERD is associated with considerably worse clinical outcomes, it remains underdiagnosed, and the exact incidence and prevalence are unknown. Fukumoto and colleagues[38] observed that 1.4% of 1786 patients who underwent left-heart catheterization had atheroembolic disease and that 64% of them were diagnosed with renal failure. One study also reported that 60% of 354 patients with atheroembolic disease were more than 70 years old, thus showing a higher occurrence in older adults.[40]

Catheter manipulations during cardiovascular procedures can disrupt the plaques, exposing the soft, cholesterol-laden core of the plaque to the arterial circulation. Administration of anticoagulants or thrombolytic therapy prevents the formation of a protective thrombus overlying an ulcerated plaque or initiates the disruption of a plaque by causing bleeding into it, thus exposing them to the hemodynamic stress of circulating blood. The embolized cholesterol crystal then lodges in small arteries, 150 to 200 nm in diameter, initiating an inflammatory reaction leading to intimal proliferation and intravascular fibrosis resulting in further

Table 1
Definitions and staging of acute kidney injury

AKI Severity/Stage	KDIGO	Serum Creatinine Criteria AKIN	RIFLE[a]	Urine Output Criteria[b]
Stage 1/Risk	Increased by ≥0.3 mg/dL within 48 h or ≥50% within 7 d	Increased by ≥0.3 mg/dL or ≥50% within 48 h	Increased by ≥1.5 times baseline	<0.5 mL/kg/h for ≥6 h
Stage 2/Injury	Increased by 2.0–2.9 times baseline	Increase by >2.0–3.0 times baseline	Increased by ≥2.0 times baseline	<0.5 mL/kg/h for 6–12 h
Stage 3/Failure	Increased ≥3.0 times baseline; or ≥0.3 mg/dL to ≥4.0 mg/dL; or KRT	Increase by >3 times baseline; or ≥0.5 mg/dL to ≥4.0 mg/dL; or on KRT	Increased by ≥3.0 times baseline or ≥0.5 mg/dL to ≥4.0 mg/dL	<0.5 mL/kg/h for ≥12 h Or <0.3 mL/kg/h for ≥24 h or anuria for ≥12 h
RIFLE Loss	—		KRT dependent for >4 wk	—
RIFLE End-stage	—		KRT dependent for >3 mo	—

Abbreviations: AKIN, acute kidney injury network; KRT, kidney replacement therapy; RIFLE, risk, injury, failure, loss, end-stage classification.
[a] Rather than a single definition and staging categories, the RIFLE classification provided definitions of AKI with increasing stringency but decreasing sensitivity (Risk, Injury, and Failure) and 2 outcome categories based on the duration of KRT-dependence (Loss and End-stage disease).
[b] Urine output criteria are identical for RIFLE, AKIN, and KDIGO.

Table 2	
Contrast-associated–acute kidney injury risk factors	
Patient-Related	**Contrast Administration Related**
Preexisting chronic kidney disease • Strongest patient-related risk factor	The osmolality of contrast medium—High osmolality agents more likely to cause CA-AKI compared with low-osmolality and iso-osmolality agents
Diabetes mellitus • Not an independent risk factor but amplified in the presence of CKD	Contrast media volume—high volume (>350 mL or >4 mL/kg) contrast administration
Hemodynamic instability	Repeat contrast administration within 72 h after the initial administration
Arteriographic procedures are higher risk than CT, owing to the delivery of more concentrated contrast material to the kidneys and the higher-risk profile of the patients getting these procedures[26]	
Advanced age	
Heart failure	

(*Adapted from* E. Schönenberger, et al. Kidney Injury after Intravenous versus Intra-arterial Contrast Agent in Patients Suspected of Having Coronary Artery Disease: A Randomized Trial. Radiology 2019;292:664-72.)

obliteration of the lumen and more ischemic changes.[41] Besides the local tissue necrosis and inflammatory response initiated by cholesterol crystals, the renin-angiotensin system and complement activation also participate in the progression of the disease.[35,42]

Hemodynamic Factors

Intraglomerular hemodynamics has an important impact on glomerular filtration rates (GFRs), peritubular capillary perfusion, and tubular function. As a highly vascular organ, kidneys receive 1.2 to 1.3 L/min of blood flow in an average adult man.[43] The blood flow is the subject of tight control by afferent arteriolar resistance variability, which is impacted by several factors, including myogenic reflex and tubuloglomerular feedback mechanisms, sympathetic nervous system, circulating vasoactive factors, endothelial nitric oxide, intrarenal angiotensin II, arachidonic acid metabolites, and paracrine systems to impact the tubuloglomerular feedback sensitivity. Consequently, the blood flow rate at the entry of glomeruli determines the intraglomerular capillary pressure and glomerular transmembrane capillary pressure gradient, which is one of the main determinants of GFR. Other determinants of glomerular transmembrane capillary pressure gradient are efferent arteriolar vascular tone, Bowman capsule pressure, glomerular membrane permeability (established by endothelial glycocalyx layer, the endothelial cell tight junctions or permeabilities, the glomerular basement membrane, and the podocyte filtration slits and slit diaphragms),

and the glomerular transmembrane capillary oncotic pressure gradient. Changes in these factors during cardiac diseases requiring interventions or due to cardiac interventions themselves could lead to a clinically relevant decline in GFR, and some cases, tubular injury, particularly when there are systemic changes in hemodynamics or local alterations in blood flow.[44]

In the peri-intervention period, systematic changes that could lead to AKI are exacerbated by cardiac dysfunction (hemodynamically relevant arrhythmias, decreased myocardial contractility, or valvular diseases). These factors could lead to reduced cardiac forward flow and increased back pressure in the kidney, causing congestion.[45] Simultaneously, local hemodynamic changes could exacerbate kidney ischemia by shunting blood flow away from the glomeruli and peritubular capillaries[46,47] by severe vasoconstriction of afferent arterioles induced by cardiorenal syndrome and exposure to contrast media or vasoactive drugs.

Apart from ischemia, volume overload, kidney congestion owing to right atrial hypertension (right ventricular failure, tricuspid valve insufficiency, pulmonary hypertension), or increased pressure around the kidney (eg, intraabdominal hypertension[48]) increases the chances of AKI.[49–52] The proposed mechanisms of AKI during kidney congestion include decreased glomerular transmembrane capillary pressure gradient owing to increased Bowman capsule pressure or increased interstitial tissue pressure leading to lower peritubular capillaries blood flow.[53]

Hydrophilic Polymer Embolism

The hydrophilic polymer is a synthetic, biodegradable coating applied to various intravascular devices and vascular grafts to reduce friction between instruments and endothelium to prevent vasospasm and thrombosis. However, the hydrophilic polymer can dislodge from these devices, resulting in downstream ischemic complications involving the brain, heart, lungs, kidneys, gastrointestinal tract, or skin.[54] This remains an underrecognized iatrogenic complication that can lead to luminal occlusion, intravascular and perivascular inflammation, and fibrous obliteration following embolism to small-, intermediate-, and large-sized vessels throughout the body.[55] Postmortem data reveal a hospital autopsy frequency of at least 13%, although the clinical incidence of polymer embolism is unknown.[55]

For clinicians, in situations wherein one encounters postprocedure embolic phenomenon, the possibility of hydrophilic polymer embolism should also be considered in addition to the usual suspects, that is, pneumatic, septic, atheromatous, thrombotic, or other foreign body embolisms.

Temporary Ventricular Support

Short-term mechanical circulatory support (MCS) devices, for example, intra-aortic balloon pump (IABP), Impella devices, and venoarterial extracorporeal membrane oxygenation (VA-ECMO), are increasingly used to support patients with cardiac failure in peri-intervention periods. However, although these devices provide hemodynamic support and improve perfusion to vital organs, their impact on kidney function remains debated.

The IABP operates through rapid cycles of diastolic inflation and systolic deflation of a helium-filled balloon in the descending aorta to enhance coronary filling and decrease afterload. IABP counterpulsation can improve forward cardiac output, renal perfusion, and coronary perfusion, potentially benefiting kidney function. However, there are also potential risks to kidney function, such as the potential for vascular site bleeding, renal artery obstruction in cases of IABP caudal migration, and atheroembolism.

Observational studies suggest that impeller-driven axial flow pumps are associated with a lower risk of AKI during high-risk PCI. Also, a study of 15 patients with cardiogenic shock found that increasing the axial flow pump rate decreased renal resistive index without changing blood pressure, suggesting kidney perfusion may have increased.[56] However, the observed increase in GFR after MCS in these studies does not appear to be sustainable. The explanations may include the profound microcirculatory compromise these patients endure before the placement of these devices, inflammatory response before and after placement of these devices, and hemolysis owing to the presence of extracorporeal circulation and pump-induced red blood cell lysis. Whether newer continuous flow devices affect kidney function differently than older pulsatile systems is under debate.[57]

The effects of venoarterial ECMO on kidney function are challenging to assess, given it is reserved for situations involving respiratory or cardiac dysfunction whereby numerous processes affecting kidney health and function are at play. Studies report the incidence of AKI in patients treated with ECMO varies from 26% to 85%. This heterogeneity is likely due to differences in patient characteristics, AKI definition criteria, and clinical settings. AKI is more common in VA-ECMO than in enovenous extracorporeal membrane oxygenation (VV-ECMO) (61% vs 46%) and is most often present on the day of ECMO cannulation.[58] The pooled estimated incidence of severe AKI requiring renal replacement therapy (RRT) in patients receiving ECMO is reported to be 45%.[59]

DIAGNOSIS

The first step in AKI diagnosis is identifying patients meeting the definition criteria. The definition of AKI has evolved over the past 20 years. The Kidney Disease: Improving Global Outcomes (KDIGO) thresholds for the presence and severity of injury are more broadly accepted.[11] AKI has also been subjected to changes in definitions and terminologies in the context of cardiovascular interventions. Table 1 summarizes the definitions of AKI based on serum creatinine and urine output criteria.[11,60,61] In addition to the current definitions of AKI, a recently concluded acute disease quality initiative consensus conference offered a definition to integrate functional and injury biomarkers for a better determination of outcome categories (Fig. 1)[62]

After identifying a patient with AKI or at high risk of AKI, conducting a diagnostic workup to identify the dominant root cause of kidney dysfunction is necessary. This workup may entail taking an appropriate medical and surgical history, a thorough and targeted physical examination, using kidney function or injury biomarkers, urinalysis, assessing hemodynamic variables, imaging, serology testing, or kidney biopsy.[63]

Biomarkers

The search for clinically applicable kidney injury or function biomarkers with improved

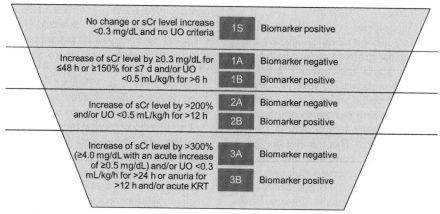

No change or sCr level increase <0.3 mg/dL and no UO criteria	1S	Biomarker positive
Increase of sCr level by ≥0.3 mg/dL for ≤48 h or ≥150% for ≤7 d and/or UO <0.5 mL/kg/h for >6 h	1A	Biomarker negative
	1B	Biomarker positive
Increase of sCr level by >200% and/or UO <0.5 mL/kg/h for >12 h	2A	Biomarker negative
	2B	Biomarker positive
Increase of sCr level by >300% (≥4.0 mg/dL with an acute increase of ≥0.5 mg/dL) and/or UO <0.3 mL/kg/h for >24 h or anuria for >12 h and/or acute KRT	3A	Biomarker negative
	3B	Biomarker positive

Fig. 1. New definition of AKI incorporating biomarkers. sCr, serum creatinine. UO, urine output; Scr, serum creatinine level.

performance compared with serum creatinine (SCr) for the early detection, diagnosis, and prognosis of AKI has proven elusive to the medical community. One has to recognize the limitations of SCr in the clinical context.[64] There is a temporal delay in the increase in SCr following an insult. In some patients, SCr elevations may not reach the threshold to qualify for AKI. Other factors, such as volume status, hemodynamic alterations, and assay variability, may significantly impact its performance. Therefore, developing and validating biomarkers for AKI in cardiovascular intervention, including CA-AKI, remain an ongoing endeavor. Multiple studies have included a modest number of patients and looked at various biomarkers. Table 3 summarizes the current landscape of the most studied kidney function and injury biomarkers.[65]

Point-of-Care Ultrasonography

The role of point-of-care ultrasonography (POCUS) examination in identifying the underlying cause of AKI in the peri-intervention period and adjusting management strategies to mitigate the impact of hemodynamic variables on AKI development is progressively recognized.[66] POCUS utilities in the peri-interventional period for AKI include but are not limited to kidney anatomy (size, echogenicity, and presence of pathologic conditions like hydronephrosis), cardiac function (systolic, diastolic, and right ventricular function, presence of tamponade, and so forth), and volume status (inferior vena cava size and collapsibility/distensibility indexes, kidney intraparenchymal venous flow pattern to detect fluid tolerance,[66] kidney elastography to assess kidney congestion,[67] lung ultrasonography,[68,69] hepatic vein flow pattern for right atrial compliance assessment, portal vein flow pattern to assess

liver congestion, and such[66]). Also, more novel contrast-enhanced ultrasonography examinations allow more information regarding renal blood flow, microvascular rarifications, and kidney congestion.[70–72]

Risk Stratification

A series of risk-stratification models incorporating patient and procedural factors has been validated in previous studies. Nevertheless, their acceptance in clinical practice has been poor owing to their essential limitations. Most studies were developed in PCI cohorts before some variables were known (eg, the volume of contrast material administered and use or nonuse of a hemodynamic-support device).[73] Examples include the original Mehran risk score, the Blue Cross Blue Shield of Michigan Cardiovascular Consortium scoring system, the ACC NCDR risk score, the Veterans Health Administration–based score, the ADVANCIS score, and the revised Mehran score.[5,31,74–76]

MANAGEMENT

Table 4 summarizes the recommendations by the National Kidney Foundation and the Society for Cardiovascular Angiography and Interventions workshop expert opinion for catheterization procedures and AKI risk prevention.[10]

Contrast-Associated–Acute Kidney Injury

Most publications on AKI in pericardiovascular intervention have focused on managing CA-AKI because of the known timing of contrast administration, defined risk factors, predictable course following contrast administration, and the prophylactic measures that may be taken beforehand to prevent its occurrence. However, recent

Table 3
Biomarkers of kidney injury and function

AKI Biomarker	Biological Role (Source)	Type of Marker (Sample)	Time of Increase After Injury	Limitations (Studied Population)
Alanine aminopeptidase, alkaline phosphatase; γ-glutamyl transpeptidase	Located in proximal tubular cells; released into urine after tubular damage[128]	Damage (urine)		Elevated in UTI, cardiovascular disease, and stroke (patients in the ICU)
Cystatin C	Produced by nucleated human cells; freely filtered[128–130]	Functional (plasma)	12–24 h after injury	Confounded by age, sex, inflammatory state, diabetes, low albumin level, muscle mass, and use of high-dose steroids (patients undergoing cardiac surgery or liver transplantation; hospitalized patients)
Hepcidin	Predominantly produced in hepatocytes; freely filtered[129]	Damage (urine and plasma)		Decreased in anemia and increased in an inflammatory state (patients undergoing cardiac surgery; patients in the ICU)
Tissue metalloproteinase-2; insulin-like growth factor binding protein-7	Metalloproteinases released during cell-cycle arrest[130–133]	Stress (urine)	As early as 4 h but typically within 12 h	Elevated in diabetes (patients undergoing cardiac or noncardiac surgery; patients in the ICU; patients in the ED)
Interleukin-18	Released into urine after tubular damage[130,134]	Damage (urine)		Elevated in an inflammatory state; lack of cutoff values (hospitalized patients; patients in the ICU or ED; patients undergoing cardiac surgery)

(continued on next page)

Table 3
(continued)

AKI Biomarker	Biological Role (Source)	Type of Marker (Sample)	Time of Increase After Injury	Limitations (Studied Population)
Kidney injury molecule-1	Produced by proximal tubular cells; released into urine after tubular damage[128–130]	Damage (urine)	12–24 h after injury	Elevated in chronic proteinuria and inflammatory diseases (hospitalized patients; patients in the ED; patients undergoing cardiac surgery; patients in the ICU)
Liver-type fatty acid-binding protein	Freely filtered and reabsorbed in proximal tubules; released into urine after tubular cell damage[129]	Damage (urine and plasma)		Associated with anemia in patients without diabetes (patients undergoing cardiac surgery; patients in the ICU or ED)
N-acetyl-β-D-glucosaminidase	Released into urine after tubular damage[128–129]	Damage (urine)	Within 2–4 h after injury	Elevated in diabetes and albuminuria (patients undergoing cardiac surgery; hospitalized patients)
Neutrophil gelatinase–associated lipocalin	At least 3 different types: (1) produced by neutrophils and epithelial tissues, including tubular cells; (2) produced by neutrophils; and (3) produced by tubular cells[128,129,134]	Damage (urine and plasma)		Elevated in sepsis, UTI, and CKD; lack of specific cutoff values (patients undergoing cardiac or noncardiac surgery; patients undergoing coronary angiography; patients in the ICU; posttransplantation patients; patients in the ED)
Proenkephalin A	Freely filtered[135]	Functional (plasma)		(Patients in the ICU; patients undergoing cardiac surgery; hospitalized patients)

Abbreviations: ED, emergency department; ICU, intensive care unit.

Table 4
Management summary for acute kidney injury prevention following cardiac interventions categorized based on the likelihood of their benefits in reducing acute kidney injury risk

Likely Beneficial	Uncertain Benefits	Unlikely Beneficial with Potential Harm
Identification of patients at risk for AKI (may be accomplished using risk prediction tools)	Diuresis in decompensated heart failure patients	Administration of N-acetylcysteine
Volume expansion in patients without decompensated heart failure	Forced diuresis with matched volume expansion	Hemofiltration or hemodialysis before or after contrast exposure
Identification of preprocedure contrast dose limits, monitoring of contrast volume administrated, and reduction in total contrast dye administration	Dilution of contrast dye with saline	Prophylactic use of adjunctive drugs (antioxidants, dopaminergic agonists, natriuretic peptides, vasopressor use in nonhypotensive patients)
Avoidance of concomitant nephrotoxins	Routine use of iso-osmolar contrast agents over low-osmolar agents	Use of sodium bicarbonate infusion
Minimization of risks for procedural complications (bleeding, hypotension, conversion to emergency surgery)	Staging of interventions or serial procedures once a contrast volume limit reached	
Transfemoral approach for TAVR	Use of technologies to limit contrast use (use of dye delivery reduction devices, automated injectors, use of noncontrast imaging tools)	
	"Zero" or ultralow contrast PCI	
	Use of radial artery access as compared with femoral artery access for coronary procedures	
	Use of biplane cine-angiography	
	Use of hemodynamic support devices as an adjunct to coronary interventions	
	Remote ischemic preconditioning	
	Carbon dioxide angiography for peripheral procedures	
	Use of high-dose HMG-CoA reductase inhibitors (statins) for kidney protection	

studies have also suggested that the previously reported risks of CA-AKI were exaggerated, and postcontrast media administration should not be the sole basis of diagnosis.[77,78] To mitigate the risk of AKI after contrast media exposure, minimizing the dose of contrast media, using low- or iso-osmolar contrast media, optimizing effective blood volume (avoid hypovolemia and hypervolemia) with hydration or diuretics, and stopping concomitant nephrotoxins are the most critical steps.

Hydration
Richard Solomon's, "Hydration to Prevent Contrast Associated Acute Kidney Injury in Patients Undergoing Cardiac Angiography," in this

issue discusses the principles, different hydration approaches, and regimens in detail. In brief, fluid administration remains the mainstay of primary prevention of CA-AKI. The theoretic rationale includes reducing vasoconstrictive hormones, natriuresis with a decrease in tubuloglomerular feedback, prevention of tubular obstruction, protection against reactive oxygen species–mediated injury, and dilution of intratubular contrast material decreasing direct tubular injury.[79,80] The practice of contrast media administration in the outpatient settings generated an interest in oral hydration. However, the studies have been inconclusive as they have limitations, including small sample size, low risk for CA-AKI, significant heterogeneity, methodologic deficiencies, oral hydration supplemented by oral sodium ingestion and IV fluids, and absence of a meaningful primary outcome.[81–85] More recent studies reported that oral hydration was as efficacious as IV fluids in less advanced CKD (estimated glomerular filtration rate [eGFR] >30 mL/min/1.73 m^2),[86,87] and larger volumes are more effective than small volumes; however, there were still concerns of confounding.[88,89]

Hydrating with IV fluids to prevent AKI following contrast exposure has been debated in the recent literature. However, the study findings were affected by including low-risk patients and cross-over to nonassigned groups. In separate meta-analyses, various fluid administration strategies were noninferior to no fluid administration in preventing CA-AKI.[90,91] It is important to note that the results of the studies that do not support IV fluid administration may be limited by the absence of participants at high risk for CA-AKI (eg, eGFR <30 mL/min).[92]

Types of fluids

In a meta-analysis of 33 RCTs comparing sodium bicarbonate solutions with isotonic saline, the conclusion was that the sodium bicarbonate significantly lowered the rate of CA-AKI (9.3% vs 12.11%; odds ratio, 0.73; 95% confidence interval [CI]: 0.56 to 0.94; $P = .01$), but there was significant intertrial heterogeneity.[93] However, the study by Mueller and colleagues[94] and PRESERVE (Prevention of Serious Adverse Events Following Angiography) trial made way for isotonic saline as the standard of care over 0.45% saline and sodium bicarbonate, respectively.[95]

Dosing of hydration

Michel and colleagues[96] compared IV fluids versus no IV fluids or only oral fluids in another meta-analysis involving 8 RCTs and 14 trials comparing intensive versus standard volume expansion. They found that intensive fluid administration was superior to standard fluid administration in preventing CA-AKI (relative risk [RR], 0.66; 95% CI: 0.52–0.85, $P = .0012$) and that IV fluids were superior to no oral hydration (RR, 0.62; 95% CI: 0.49–0.77, $P<.001$).

Hemodynamically guided tailored fluid administration has been an attractive approach owing to risks associated with volume overload in patients at moderate to high risk of developing CA-AKI. The left ventricular end-diastolic pressure (LVEDP), central venous pressure, and bioimpedance vector analysis are a few of the assessment parameters that have been used to guide the dosing of fluids, and most of these have been shown to be superior to standard fluid administration.[97–100]

Broad recommendations for hydration

Broad recommendations for hydration, based on these data, for patients at risk of CA-AKI undergoing coronary angiography and other vascular interventions include the following[92]:

1. IV fluid is superior to prescribing no fluids, particularly in patients with eGFR less than 45 mL/min/1.73 m^2,
2. In patients with eGFRs of 45 to 59 mL/min/1.73 m^2 with multiple risk factors, it would be reasonable to administer IV fluids, although the evidence is not robust,
3. Current literature supports IV isotonic saline over more hypotonic IV solutions, and isotonic sodium bicarbonate,
4. Additional data are needed before any recommendations can be made regarding the duration of fluid administration, oral hydration, hemodynamics-guided fluid administration, or forced diuresis with matched IV replacement fluids,
5. Excessive use of IV fluids among those with volume overload, heart failure, kidney dysfunction, and respiratory failure should be avoided.

Nonetheless, contrast agents have evolved, and other preventive measures have led to lower AKI rates after contrast material administration.[77,101–103] Similar studies are important to reassure clinicians to proceed with required interventional procedures if otherwise indicated and not deprive patients of appropriate care in the presence of CKD and other risk factors, a phenomenon described as "Renalism."[104]

Type of contrast media

Contrast agents are classified based on their osmolarity (Table 5). The most commonly used

Table 5
Contrast media molecular characteristics

Osmolarity	High	Low	Low	Iso-Osmolar
Osmolarity (mOsm/kg H_2O)	1551	600	413–796	290
Ionicity	Ionic	Ionic	Nonionic	Nonionic
Number of benzoate rings	Monomer	Dimer	Monomer	Dimer
Name	Diatrizoate meglumine Diatrizoate sodium	Ioxaglate meglumine Ioxaglate sodium	Iohexol Iopamidol Ioversol Iopromide	Iodixanol
Contrast concentration (mg/mL)	760	589	408–755	550–652
Iodine concentration (mg/mL)	370	320	200–370	270–320
Viscosity at 37°C (mPa.s)	11	8	2–10	6–12

contrast agents are among low- or iso-osmolar agents, favored over the high-osmolar media. There is no clear consensus about the benefit of iso-osmolar over low-osmolar contrast agents or the superiority of any single agent among the low-osmolar and iso-osmolar agents.[105–107] Studies have, however, supported the role of iso-osmolar contrast media in preventing limb pain during peripheral angiography and the potential reduction in composite renal and cardiovascular events.[108–110]

Contrast media volume

Studies have consistently demonstrated a direct dose-response relationship between the volume of contrast administered and the incidence of AKI.[111,112] Among the many proposed contrast dose limits in the literature, the total contrast volume indexed to estimate kidney function provides a validated ratio for determining the

limit.[111,113,114] In practice, one should be attentive to baseline kidney function, meticulously plan cases, hold discussions with teams, and monitor the volume of intraprocedural dye to achieve the lowest contrast volume used. The most recent recommendations regarding the use of the race-free 2021 Chronic Kidney Disease Epidemiology Collaboration equation should be the one to be used to obtain calculated eGFR and plan the contrast volume to be administered.[115] Although the cardiology-based guidelines have recommended a contrast volume to eGFR ratio of 3.7[116] as an upper dose limit, multiple studies demonstrate that risk increases substantially at lower thresholds; therefore, a ratio of 2:3 may be preferred.[117] A recently published study looked at the effect of clinical decision support with audit and feedback on preventing AKI in patients undergoing coronary angiography. In the stepped-wedge, cluster

Table 6
Management approach for patients with chronic kidney disease undergoing cardiovascular interventions

Before Intervention Care	During Intervention Care	After Procedure Care
AKI risk evaluation	Monitor contrast volume	Close clinical follow-up
Avoid nephrotoxins	Limit total contrast volume	Monitor changes in serum creatinine
IV crystalloids for non-volume-overloaded patients	Minimize bleeding risk	Optimize cardiac medications
Calculate contrast volume limit	Avoid hypotension	Follow up with nephrology
Consider nephrology consultation for high-risk patients	Measure LVEDP	
	Adjust volume expansion as needed	
	Stage interventions if appropriate	

Abbreviation: LVEDP, left ventricular end-diastolic pressure.

RCT conducted in Alberta, Canada, that included 34 cardiologists who performed 7820 procedures, the incidence of AKI during the intervention period compared with the control period was 7.2% versus 8.6%, with a time-adjusted absolute risk reduction of 2.3%, a statistically significant difference.[9]

Avoidance of nephrotoxins

Although nephrotoxic medications should be avoided in patients at risk of developing AKI, it must be emphasized that most patients undergoing cardiovascular interventions are at a higher risk because of either the presence of preexisting CKD or hemodynamic status, arteriographic procedure, or comorbidities, such as heart failure and diabetes mellitus. Particularly, drugs that could lead to higher afferent arteriolar vasoconstriction of lower glomerular transmembrane capillary pressure gradient, for example, nonsteroidal anti-inflammatory agents, angiotensin-converting-enzyme inhibitors, or angiotensin-receptor blockers, and nephrotoxic antibiotics like amphotericin B or vancomycin, should be avoided. In addition, the diuretic administration should be individualized according to the clinical scenario and the volume status of patients.

The increase of SCr and drop in eGFR is known to occur with the use of renin angiotensin system blockers and sodium-glucose cotransporter-2 inhibitors secondary to largely transient hemodynamic changes in blood flow. The studies regarding their use during the peri-intervention period have been inconclusive.[118–120] However, one should pay close attention to the risk of failure to resume these drugs after the intervention, which are beneficial for the long-term management of CKD and CHF.

Table 6 describes the preventive measures that should be considered before, during, or after cardiac interventions to reduce the risk of AKI.

Atheroembolic Disease, Management

Box 1 provides a summary of risk stratification and management of AERD. Management of AERD remains primarily supportive, and no specific therapy exists for the condition. Performance of further invasive diagnostic/therapeutic vascular interventional procedures or surgery should be avoided or postponed if possible. Anticoagulant therapy should be stopped after carefully considering the clinical context. Blood pressure control and management of congestive heart failure remain critical in this condition. Some patients may develop bowel ischemia in severe cases necessitating parenteral nutrition for adequate nutrition.

Box 1
Risk stratification and management of atheroembolic renal disease

Population at risk for atheroembolic renal disease

- Male sex
- Age greater than 60 years
- White race
- Hypertension
- Tobacco use
- Diabetes mellitus
- Atherosclerotic vascular disease
  - Ischemic cardiac disease
  - Cerebrovascular disease
  - Abdominal aortic aneurysm
  - Peripheral vascular disease
  - Ischemic nephropathy

Treatment of atheroembolic renal disease

- Goal
  - Restrict extent of the ischemic damage
  - Prevent recurrent embolization
- No definitive treatment has been established
- Therapeutic modalities are mostly preventive and supportive
- Avoid further precipitating events
  - Withdrawal of anticoagulant therapy
  - Avoid any new radiologic or aortic surgery procedure
- Medical intervention
  - Mostly symptomatic
  - Aggressive treatment of associated hypertension and heart and kidney failure
- Kidney replacement therapy if clinically indicated
- Adequate nutritional support when needed; pay attention to bowel ischemia
- Steroids in patients with multisystem involvement and recurrent, progressive disease
- Statins should be offered to all patients with atheroembolic renal disease

---

Corticosteroid therapy for reducing the inflammatory response remains controversial, with some studies showing benefits,[121–123] whereas others reveal no effect on renal or patient outcomes.[40] Statins have been found to have beneficial effects in multiple observational studies.[40,124–126] This has been attributed to plaque stabilization and regression through lipid-lowering and anti-inflammatory mechanisms.

Removal of the source of emboli surgically, although proposed as a definitive treatment, is often not possible because of the complexity of the vascular disease, leading to a higher risk of further embolization and patients' general frailty. Keen and colleagues[127] examined the surgical approach in a prospective study involving 100 patients. They found that surgery can be an option when the emboli source is in the infrarenal aorta. The increased morbidity and mortality in patients with suprarenal aortic pathologic condition are due to the risk for visceral and renal atheroembolization. Nonetheless, surgical intervention should be regarded as rescue therapy and restricted to life-threatening situations.

Kidney replacement therapy for uremia and fluid management may be required for patients with diuretic-refractory oliguria or volume overload. In addition, some studies advocate using peritoneal dialysis, citing the nonrequirement of anticoagulation as an advantage over hemodialysis. However, hemodialysis without or with minimal anticoagulation is acceptable as well.[35]

SUMMARY

AKI following cardiac interventions is common and is associated with dire consequences. It is often due to multiple pathophysiologic mechanisms, which makes the diagnostic and workup approach challenging. Meanwhile, the incidence and severity of AKI following cardiac interventions could be mitigated with appropriate preventive measures. Therefore, a multidisciplinary team comprising nephrologists, pharmacists, nurses, and cardiologists is needed to manage postinterventional AKI.

CLINICS CARE POINTS

- Optimal risk stratification using risk prediction tools, hemodynamic optimization, and a multidisciplinary collaborative approach is essential to preventing acute kidney injury in the pericardiovascular intervention period.
- Optimization of volume status, minimization of contrast volume, and avoidance of concomitant nephrotoxins lower the incidence of acute kidney injury.
- Incorporation of biomarkers for diagnosis of acute kidney injury and point-of-care ultrasound to facilitate fluid management are likely to benefit this at-risk population.

- Once acute kidney injury has been established, kidney replacement therapy should be used to support the patient's hemodynamics and fluid and electrolyte status.

CONFLICT OF INTEREST

None of the authors have any conflict of interest to report.

FINANCIAL SUPPORT

No financial support was used for the preparation of this article.

REFERENCES

1. McCullough PA, Adam A, Becker CR, et al. Epidemiology and prognostic implications of contrast-induced nephropathy. Am J Cardiol 2006;98(6a): 5k–13k.
2. Ram P, Horn B, Lo KBU, et al. Acute Kidney Injury Post Cardiac Catheterization: Does Vascular Access Route Matter? Curr Cardiol Rev 2019;15(2): 96–101.
3. Sardinha DM, Simor A, de Oliveira Moura LD, et al. Risk Factors for Acute Renal Failure after Cardiac Catheterization Most Cited in the Literature: An Integrative Review. Int J Environ Res Public Health 2020;17(10). https://doi.org/10.3390/ijerph17103392.
4. Silver SA, Chertow GM. The Economic Consequences of Acute Kidney Injury. Nephron 2017; 137(4):297–301.
5. Tsai TT, Patel UD, Chang TI, et al. Validated contemporary risk model of acute kidney injury in patients undergoing percutaneous coronary interventions: insights from the National Cardiovascular Data Registry Cath-PCI Registry. J Am Heart Assoc. Dec 2014;3(6):e001380.
6. Safley DM, Salisbury AC, Tsai TT, et al. Acute Kidney Injury Following In-Patient Lower Extremity Vascular Intervention: From the National Cardiovascular Data Registry. JACC Cardiovasc Interv 2021;14(3):333–41.
7. Grossman PM, Ali SS, Aronow HD, et al. Contrast-induced nephropathy in patients undergoing endovascular peripheral vascular intervention: Incidence, risk factors, and outcomes as observed in the Blue Cross Blue Shield of Michigan Cardiovascular Consortium. J Interv Cardiol 2017;30(3): 274–80.
8. Julien HM, Stebbins A, Vemulapalli S, et al. Incidence, predictors, and outcomes of acute kidney injury in patients undergoing transcatheter aortic valve replacement: insights from the Society of

Thoracic Surgeons/American College of Cardiology National Cardiovascular Data Registry–Transcatheter Valve Therapy Registry. Circulation: Cardiovascular Interventions 2021;14(4):e010032.

9. James MT, Har BJ, Tyrrell BD, et al. Effect of Clinical Decision Support With Audit and Feedback on Prevention of Acute Kidney Injury in Patients Undergoing Coronary Angiography: A Randomized Clinical Trial. JAMA 2022;328(9):839–49.

10. Prasad A, Palevsky PM, Bansal S, et al. Management of Patients With Kidney Disease in Need of Cardiovascular Catheterization: A Scientific Workshop Cosponsored by the National Kidney Foundation and the Society for Cardiovascular Angiography and Interventions. Journal of the Society for Cardiovascular Angiography & Interventions 2022;1(6):100445.

11. Section 2: AKI Definition. Kidney Int Suppl 2012;2(1):19–36.

12. Mehran R, Dangas GD, Weisbord SD. Contrast-Associated Acute Kidney Injury. N Engl J Med 2019;380(22):2146–55.

13. Cho E, Ko G-J. The Pathophysiology and the Management of Radiocontrast-Induced Nephropathy. Diagnostics 2022;12(1):180.

14. Clark EG, James MT, Hiremath S, et al. Predictive Models for Kidney Recovery and Death in Patients Continuing Dialysis as Outpatients after Starting In Hospital. Clin J Am Soc Nephrol 2023. https://doi.org/10.2215/CJN.0000000000000173.

15. Andreucci M, Fuiano G, Presta P, et al. Radiocontrast media cause dephosphorylation of Akt and downstream signaling targets in human renal proximal tubular cells. Biochem Pharmacol 2006;72(10):1334–42.

16. Dangas G, Iakovou I, Nikolsky E, et al. Contrast-induced nephropathy after percutaneous coronary interventions in relation to chronic kidney disease and hemodynamic variables. Am J Cardiol 2005;95(1):13–9.

17. Cashion W, Weisbord SD. Radiographic Contrast Media and the Kidney. Clin J Am Soc Nephrol 2022. https://doi.org/10.2215/cjn.16311221. CJN.16311221.

18. Sun Moon K, Ran-hui C, Jung Pyo L, et al. Incidence and Outcomes of Contrast-Induced Nephropathy After Computed Tomography in Patients With CKD: A Quality Improvement Report. Am J Kidney Dis 2010;55(6):1018–25.

19. McCullough PA, Wolyn R, Rocher LL, et al. Acute renal failure after coronary intervention: incidence, risk factors, and relationship to mortality. Am J Med 1997;103(5):368–75.

20. Berns AS. Nephrotoxicity of contrast media. Kidney Int 1989;36(4):730–40.

21. Erley C. Concomitant drugs with exposure to contrast media. Kidney Int Suppl 2006;(100):S20–4.

22. Cigarroa RG, Lange RA, Williams RH, et al. Dosing of contrast material to prevent contrast nephropathy in patients with renal disease. Am J Med 1989;86(6 Pt 1):649–52.

23. Davidson C, Stacul F, McCullough PA, et al. Contrast medium use. Am J Cardiol 2006;98(6a):42k–58k.

24. Cichoń M, Wybraniec MT, Okoń O, et al. Repeated Dose of Contrast Media and the Risk of Contrast-Induced Acute Kidney Injury in a Broad Population of Patients Hospitalized in Cardiology Department. J Clin Med 2023;12(6). https://doi.org/10.3390/jcm12062166.

25. Freeman RV, O'Donnell M, Share D, et al. Nephropathy requiring dialysis after percutaneous coronary intervention and the critical role of an adjusted contrast dose. Am J Cardiol 2002;90(10):1068–73.

26. Schönenberger E, Martus P, Bosserdt M, et al. Kidney Injury after Intravenous versus Intra-arterial Contrast Agent in Patients Suspected of Having Coronary Artery Disease: A Randomized Trial. Radiology 2019;292(3):664–72.

27. Kooiman J, Le Haen PA, Gezgin G, et al. Contrast-induced acute kidney injury and clinical outcomes after intra-arterial and intravenous contrast administration: Risk comparison adjusted for patient characteristics by design. Am Heart J 2013;165(5):793–9.e1.

28. McDonald JS, Leake CB, McDonald RJ, et al. Acute Kidney Injury After Intravenous Versus Intra-Arterial Contrast Material Administration in a Paired Cohort. Invest Radiol 2016;51(12):804–9.

29. Karlsberg RP, Dohad SY, Sheng R. Iodixanol Peripheral Computed Tomographic Angiography Study Investigator P. Contrast medium-induced acute kidney injury: comparison of intravenous and intraarterial administration of iodinated contrast medium. J Vasc Interv Radiol. Aug 2011;22(8):1159–65.

30. Chaudhury P, Armanyous S, Harb SC, et al. Intra-Arterial versus Intravenous Contrast and Renal Injury in Chronic Kidney Disease: A Propensity-Matched Analysis. Nephron 2019;141(1):31–40.

31. Mehran R, Aymong ED, Nikolsky E, et al. A simple risk score for prediction of contrast-induced nephropathy after percutaneous coronary intervention: development and initial validation. J Am Coll Cardiol 2004;44(7):1393–9.

32. Mo H, Ye F, Chen D, et al. A Predictive Model Based on a New CI-AKI Definition to Predict Contrast Induced Nephropathy in Patients With Coronary Artery Disease With Relatively Normal Renal Function. Front Cardiovasc Med 2021;8:762576.

33. Petek BJ, Bravo PE, Kim F, et al. Incidence and Risk Factors for Postcontrast Acute Kidney Injury

in Survivors of Sudden Cardiac Arrest. Ann Emerg Med 2016;67(4):469–76.e1.

34. Seibert FS, Heringhaus A, Pagonas N, et al. Biomarkers in the prediction of contrast media induced nephropathy - the BITCOIN study. PLoS One 2020;15(7):e0234921.

35. Scolari F, Ravani P. Atheroembolic renal disease. Lancet 2010;375(9726):1650–60.

36. Cappiello RA, Espinoza LR, Adelman H, et al. Cholesterol embolism: a pseudovasculitic syndrome. Semin Arthritis Rheum. May 1989;18(4):240–6.

37. Modi KS, Rao VK. Atheroembolic renal disease. J Am Soc Nephrol. Aug 2001;12(8):1781–7.

38. Fukumoto Y, Tsutsui H, Tsuchihashi M, et al. The incidence and risk factors of cholesterol embolization syndrome, a complication of cardiac catheterization: a prospective study. J Am Coll Cardiol 2003;42(2):211–6.

39. Mittal BV, Alexander MP, Rennke HG, et al. Atheroembolic renal disease: a silent masquerader. Kidney Int 2008;73(1):126–30.

40. Scolari F, Ravani P, Gaggi R, et al. The challenge of diagnosing atheroembolic renal disease: clinical features and prognostic factors. Circulation 2007;116(3):298–304.

41. Saric M, Kronzon I. Cholesterol embolization syndrome. Curr Opin Cardiol. Nov 2011;26(6):472–9.

42. Scoble JE, O'Donnell PJ. Renal atheroembolic disease: the Cinderella of nephrology? Nephrol Dial Transplant. Aug 1996;11(8):1516–7.

43. Yu ASL, Chertow GM, Luyckx VA, et al. Brenner & rector's the kidney. Amsterdam, The Netherlands: Elsevier; 2020.

44. Sharfuddin AA, Molitoris BA. Pathophysiology of ischemic acute kidney injury. Nat Rev Nephrol 2011;7(4):189–200.

45. Vahdatpour C, Collins D, Goldberg S. Cardiogenic Shock. J Am Heart Assoc 2019;8(8):e011991.

46. Casellas D, Mimran A. Aglomerular pathways in intrarenal microvasculature of aged rats. Am J Anat 1979;156(2):293–9.

47. Casellas D, Mimran A. Shunting in renal microvasculature of the rat: a scanning electron microscopic study of corrosion casts. Anat Rec 1981;201(2):237–48.

48. Dalfino L, Tullo L, Donadio I, et al. Intra-abdominal hypertension and acute renal failure in critically ill patients. Intensive Care Med 2008;34(4):707–13.

49. Kim IY, Kim JH, Lee DW, et al. Fluid overload and survival in critically ill patients with acute kidney injury receiving continuous renal replacement therapy. PLoS One 2017;12(2):e0172137.

50. Woodward CW, Lambert J, Ortiz-Soriano V, et al. Fluid Overload Associates With Major Adverse Kidney Events in Critically Ill Patients With Acute Kidney Injury Requiring Continuous Renal Replacement Therapy. Critical care medicine. Sep 2019;47(9):e753–60.

51. Biancofiore G, Bindi L, Romanelli AM, et al. Renal failure and abdominal hypertension after liver transplantation: determination of critical intra-abdominal pressure. Liver Transpl 2002;8(12):1175–81.

52. Mullens W, Abrahams Z, Skouri HN, et al. Elevated intra-abdominal pressure in acute decompensated heart failure: a potential contributor to worsening renal function? J Am Coll Cardiol 2008;51(3):300–6.

53. Juncos LA, Wieruszewski PM, Kashani K. Pathophysiology of Acute Kidney Injury in Critical Illness: A Narrative Review. Compr Physiol. Sep 8 2022;12(4):3767–80.

54. Kudose S, Adomako EA, D'Agati VD, et al. Collapsing Glomerulopathy Associated With Hydrophilic Polymer Emboli. Kidney Int Rep. Apr 2019;4(4):619–23.

55. Mehta RI, Mehta RI. Hydrophilic Polymer Embolism: An Update for Physicians. Am J Med 2017-07-01 2017;130(7):e287–90.

56. Lemaire A, Anderson MB, Lee LY, et al. The Impella device for acute mechanical circulatory support in patients in cardiogenic shock. Ann Thorac Surg. Jan 2014;97(1):133–8.

57. Sandner SE, Zimpfer D, Zrunek P, et al. Renal function after implantation of continuous versus pulsatile flow left ventricular assist devices. J Heart Lung Transplant 2008;27(5):469–73.

58. Delmas C, Zapetskaia T, Conil JM, et al. 3-month prognostic impact of severe acute renal failure under veno-venous ECMO support: Importance of time of onset. J Crit Care 2018;44:63–71.

59. Thongprayoon C, Lertjitbanjong P, Hansrivijit P, et al. Acute Kidney Injury in Patients Undergoing Cardiac Transplantation: A Meta-Analysis. Medicines 2019;6(4):108.

60. Bellomo R, Ronco C, Kellum JA, et al. Acute renal failure - definition, outcome measures, animal models, fluid therapy and information technology needs: the Second International Consensus Conference of the Acute Dialysis Quality Initiative (ADQI) Group. Crit Care 2004;8(4):R204–12.

61. Mehta RL, Kellum JA, Shah SV, et al. Acute Kidney Injury Network: report of an initiative to improve outcomes in acute kidney injury. Crit Care 2007;11(2):R31.

62. Ostermann M, Zarbock A, Goldstein S, et al. Recommendations on Acute Kidney Injury Biomarkers From the Acute Disease Quality Initiative Consensus Conference: A Consensus Statement. JAMA Netw Open 2020;3(10):e2019209.

63. Kashani K, Rosner MH, Haase M, et al. Quality Improvement Goals for Acute Kidney Injury. Clin J Am Soc Nephrol 2019;14(6):941–53.

64. Kashani K, Rosner MH, Ostermann M. Creatinine: From physiology to clinical application. Eur J Intern Med 2020;72:9–14.

65. Levin D, Bansal S, Prasad A. The Role of Novel Cardiorenal Biomarkers in the Cardiac Catheterization Laboratory for the Detection of Acute Kidney Injury. Rev Cardiovasc Med 2016;17(3–4): 100–14.

66. Coca SG, Yalavarthy R, Concato J, et al. Biomarkers for the diagnosis and risk stratification of acute kidney injury: A systematic review. Kidney Int 2008;73(9):1008–16.

67. Ho J, Tangri N, Komenda P, et al. Urinary, Plasma, and Serum Biomarkers' Utility for Predicting Acute Kidney Injury Associated With Cardiac Surgery in Adults: A Meta-analysis. Am J Kidney Dis 2015; 66(6):993–1005.

68. Kane-Gill SL, Meersch M, Bell M. Biomarker-guided management of acute kidney injury. Curr Opin Crit Care 2020;26(6):556–62.

69. Yang HS, Hur M, Lee KR, et al. Biomarker Rule-in or Rule-out in Patients With Acute Diseases for Validation of Acute Kidney Injury in the Emergency Department (BRAVA): A Multicenter Study Evaluating Urinary TIMP-2/IGFBP7. Annals of Laboratory Medicine 2022;42(2):178–87.

70. Ostermann M, McCullough PA, Forni LG, et al. Kinetics of Urinary Cell Cycle Arrest Markers for Acute Kidney Injury Following Exposure to Potential Renal Insults. Crit Care Med 2018;46(3):375–83.

71. Kashani K, Al-Khafaji A, Ardiles T, et al. Discovery and validation of cell cycle arrest biomarkers in human acute kidney injury. Crit Care 2013;17(1): R25.

72. Charlton JR, Portilla D, Okusa MD. A basic science view of acute kidney injury biomarkers. Nephrol Dial Transplant 2014;29(7):1301–11.

73. Legrand M, Hollinger A, Vieillard-Baron A, et al. One-Year Prognosis of Kidney Injury at Discharge From the ICU: A Multicenter Observational Study. Crit Care Med 2019;47(12):e953–61.

74. Safadi S, Murthi S, Kashani KB. Use of Ultrasound to Assess Hemodynamics in Acutely Ill Patients. Kidney360 2021;2(8):1349–59.

75. Kashani KB, Mao SA, Safadi S, et al. Association between kidney intracapsular pressure and ultrasound elastography. journal article. Crit Care. 2017;21(1):251.

76. Lichtenstein DA, Meziere GA. Relevance of lung ultrasound in the diagnosis of acute respiratory failure: the BLUE protocol. Chest. Jul 2008; 134(1):117–25.

77. Lichtenstein DA, Meziere GA, Lagoueyte JF, et al. A-lines and B-lines: lung ultrasound as a bedside tool for predicting pulmonary artery occlusion pressure in the critically ill. Chest 2009;136(4): 1014–20.

78. Schneider AG, Hofmann L, Wuerzner G, et al. Renal perfusion evaluation with contrast-enhanced ultrasonography. Nephrol Dial Transplant 2011;27(2):674–81.

79. Schneider AG, Goodwin MD, Schelleman A, et al. Contrast-enhanced ultrasonography to evaluate changes in renal cortical microcirculation induced by noradrenaline: a pilot study. Crit Care 2014; 18(6):653.

80. Wang L, Mohan C. Contrast-enhanced ultrasound: A promising method for renal microvascular perfusion evaluation. J Transl Int Med 2016; 4(3):104–8.

81. Mehran R, Dangas GD, Weisbord SD. Contrast-Associated Acute Kidney Injury. N Engl J Med 2019-05-30 2019;380(22):2146–55.

82. Mehran R, Owen R, Chiarito M, et al. A contemporary simple risk score for prediction of contrast-associated acute kidney injury after percutaneous coronary intervention: derivation and validation from an observational registry. Lancet 2021; 398(10315). 1974-19.

83. Gurm HS, Seth M, Kooiman J, et al. A novel tool for reliable and accurate prediction of renal complications in patients undergoing percutaneous coronary intervention. J Am Coll Cardiol 2013; 61(22):2242–8.

84. Brown JR, MacKenzie TA, Maddox TM, et al. Acute kidney injury risk prediction in patients undergoing coronary angiography in a national veterans health administration cohort with external validation. Article. J Am Heart Assoc 2015;4(12): e002136.

85. McDonald JS, McDonald RJ, Comin J, et al. Frequency of acute kidney injury following intravenous contrast medium administration: a systematic review and meta-analysis. Radiology 2013;267(1):119–28.

86. Davenport MS, Perazella MA, Yee J, et al. Use of intravenous iodinated contrast media in patients with kidney disease: consensus statements from the American College of Radiology and the National Kidney Foundation. Radiology 2020;294(3):660–8.

87. Trivedi HS, Moore H, Nasr S, et al. A randomized prospective trial to assess the role of saline hydration on the development of contrast nephrotoxicity. Nephron Clin Pract 2003;93(1):c29–34.

88. Cho R, Javed N, Traub D, et al. Oral hydration and alkalinization is noninferior to intravenous therapy for prevention of contrast-induced nephropathy in patients with chronic kidney disease. J Interv Cardiol 2010;23(5).

89. Martin-Moreno PL, Varo N, Martínez-Ansó E, et al. Comparison of intravenous and oral hydration in the prevention of contrast-induced acute kidney injury in low-risk patients: a randomized trial. Nephron 2015;131(1):51–8.

90. Cheungpasitporn W, Thongprayoon C, Brabec BA, et al. Oral hydration for prevention of contrast-induced acute kidney injury in elective radiological procedures: a systematic review and meta-analysis of randomized controlled trials. N Am J Med Sci 2014;6(12):618.

91. Hiremath S, Akbari A, Shabana W, et al. Prevention of contrast-induced acute kidney injury: is simple oral hydration similar to intravenous? A systematic review of the evidence. PLoS One 2013;8(3):e60009.

92. Sebastià C, Páez-Carpio A, Guillen E, et al. Oral hydration compared to intravenous hydration in the prevention of post-contrast acute kidney injury in patients with chronic kidney disease stage IIIb: A phase III non-inferiority study (NICIR study). Eur J Radiol 2021;136:109509.

93. Wee NK, Tiong SC, Lee CH, et al. Safety of a rapid outpatient hydration protocol for patients with renal impairment requiring intravenous iodinated contrast media for computed tomography. Singapore Med J 2021;62(11):588.

94. Song F, Sun G, Liu J, et al. The association between post-procedural oral hydration and risk of contrast-induced acute kidney injury among ST-elevation myocardial infarction patients undergoing primary percutaneous coronary intervention. Ann Transl Med 2019;7(14).

95. Xie W, Zhou Y, Liao Z, et al. Effect of Oral Hydration on Contrast-Induced Acute Kidney Injury among Patients after Primary Percutaneous Coronary Intervention. Cardiorenal Med 2021;11(5–6):243–51.

96. Sterling KA, Tehrani T, Rudnick MR. Clinical significance and preventive strategies for contrast-induced nephropathy. Curr Opin Nephrol Hypertens 2008; 17(6):616–23.

97. Erley CM. Does hydration prevent radiocontrast-induced acute renal failure? Nephrology, dialysis, transplantation. official publication of the European Dialysis and Transplant Association-European Renal Association 1999;14(5):1064–6.

98. Wang Z, Song Y, Li Y. Role of hydration in contrast-induced nephropathy in patients who underwent primary percutaneous coronary intervention a meta-analysis of randomized trials. Int Heart J 2019;60(5):1077–82.

99. Cai Q, Jing R, Zhang W, et al. Hydration strategies for preventing contrast-induced acute kidney injury: a systematic review and bayesian network meta-analysis. J Interv Cardiol 2020;2020.

100. Michel P, Amione-Guerra J, Sheikh O, et al. Meta-analysis of intravascular volume expansion strategies to prevent contrast-associated acute kidney injury following invasive angiography. Catheter Cardiovasc Interv 2021;98(6):1120–32.

101. Rudnick MR, Fay K, Wahba IM. Fluid administration strategies for the prevention of contrast-associated acute kidney injury. Curr Opin Nephrol Hypertens 2022;31(5):414–24.

102. Mueller C, Buerkle G, Buettner HJ, et al. Prevention of contrast media–associated nephropathy: randomized comparison of 2 hydration regimens in 1620 patients undergoing coronary angioplasty. Arch Intern Med 2002;162(3):329–36.

103. Ali-Hassan-Sayegh S, Mirhosseini SJ, Ghodratipour Z, et al. Strategies preventing contrast-induced nephropathy after coronary angiography: a comprehensive meta-analysis and systematic review of 125 randomized controlled trials. Angiology 2017;68(5):389–413.

104. Weisbord SD, Gallagher M, Jneid H, et al. Outcomes after angiography with sodium bicarbonate and acetylcysteine. N Engl J Med 2018; 378(7):603–14.

105. Brar SS, Aharonian V, Mansukhani P, et al. Haemodynamic-guided fluid administration for the prevention of contrast-induced acute kidney injury: the POSEIDON randomised controlled trial. Lancet 2014;383(9931):1814–23.

106. Marashizadeh A, Sanati HR, Sadeghipour P, et al. Left ventricular end-diastolic pressure-guided hydration for the prevention of contrast-induced acute kidney injury in patients with stable ischemic heart disease: the LAKESIDE trial. Int Urol Nephrol 2019;51:1815–22.

107. Qian G, Fu Z, Guo J, et al. Prevention of contrast-induced nephropathy by central venous pressure–guided fluid administration in chronic kidney disease and congestive heart failure patients. JACC Cardiovasc Interv 2016;9(1):89–96.

108. Maioli M, Toso A, Leoncini M, et al. Bio-impedance-guided hydration for the prevention of contrast-induced kidney injury: the HYDRA study. J Am Coll Cardiol 2018;71(25):2880–9.

109. Bartels ED, Brun G, Gammeltoft A, et al. Acute Annria following intravenous pyelography in a patient with myelomatosis. Acta Med Scand 1954; 150(4):297–302.

110. Killmann SA, Gjørup S, Thaysen JH. Fatal acute renal failure following intravenous pyelography in a patient with multiple myeloma. Acta Med Scand 1957;158(1):43–6.

111. Weisbord SD, Mor MK, Resnick AL, et al. Prevention, incidence, and outcomes of contrast-induced acute kidney injury. Arch Intern Med 2008;168(12): 1325–32.

112. Chertow GM, Normand S-LT, McNeil BJ. "Renalism": Inappropriately Low Rates of Coronary Angiography in Elderly Individuals with Renal Insufficiency. J Am Soc Nephrol 2004;15(9): 2462–8.

113. Reed M, Meier P, Tamhane UU, et al. The Relative Renal Safety of Iodixanol Compared With Low-Osmolar Contrast Media: A Meta-Analysis of

Randomized Controlled Trials. JACC Cardiovasc Interv 2009;2(7):645–54.

114. McCullough PA, Bertrand ME, Brinker JA, et al. A Meta-Analysis of the Renal Safety of Isosmolar Iodixanol Compared With Low-Osmolar Contrast Media. J Am Coll Cardiol 2006;48(4):692–9.

115. Heinrich MC, Häberle L, Müller V, et al. Nephrotoxicity of Iso-osmolar Iodixanol Compared with Nonionic Low-osmolar Contrast Media: Meta-analysis of Randomized Controlled Trials. Radiology 2009;250(1):68–86.

116. Palena LM, Sacco ZD, Brigato C, et al. Discomfort assessment in peripheral angiography: Randomized clinical trial of Iodixanol 270 versus Ioversol 320 in diabetics with critical limb ischemia. Catheter Cardiovasc Interv 2014;84(6):1019–25.

117. Prasad A, Amin AP, Ryan MP, et al. Use of iso-osmolar contrast media during endovascular revascularization is associated with a lower incidence of major adverse renal, cardiac, or limb events. Catheter Cardiovasc Interv 2022;99(4):1335–42.

118. Amin AP, Prasad A, Ryan MP, et al. Association of Iso-Osmolar vs Low-Osmolar Contrast Media With Major Adverse Renal or Cardiovascular Events in Patients at High Risk for Acute Kidney Injury Undergoing Endovascular Abdominal Aortic Aneurysm Repair. Article. J Invasive Cardiol 2021;33(8):E640–6.

119. Gurm HS, Dixon SR, Smith DE, et al. Renal Function-Based Contrast Dosing to Define Safe Limits of Radiographic Contrast Media in Patients Undergoing Percutaneous Coronary Interventions. J Am Coll Cardiol 2011;58(9):907–14.

120. Amin AP, Bach RG, Caruso ML, et al. Association of Variation in Contrast Volume With Acute Kidney Injury in Patients Undergoing Percutaneous Coronary Intervention. JAMA Cardiology 2017;2(9):1007–12.

121. Cigarroa RG, Lange RA, Williams RH, et al. Dosing of contrast material to prevent contrast nephropathy in patients with renal disease. Am J Med 1989;86(6):649–52.

122. Laskey WK, Jenkins C, Selzer F, et al. Volume-to-Creatinine Clearance Ratio: A Pharmacokinetically Based Risk Factor for Prediction of Early Creatinine Increase After Percutaneous Coronary Intervention. J Am Coll Cardiol 2007;50(7):584–90.

123. Delgado C, Baweja M, Crews DC, et al. A Unifying Approach for GFR Estimation: Recommendations of the NKF-ASN Task Force on Reassessing the Inclusion of Race in Diagnosing Kidney Disease. Am J Kidney Dis 2022;79(2):268–88.e1.

124. Mager A, Vaknin Assa H, Lev EI, et al. The ratio of contrast volume to glomerular filtration rate predicts outcomes after percutaneous coronary intervention for ST-segment elevation acute myocardial infarction. Catheter Cardiovasc Interv 2011;78(2):198–201.

125. Kooiman J, Seth M, Share D, et al. The Association between Contrast Dose and Renal Complications Post PCI across the Continuum of Procedural Estimated Risk. PLoS One 2014;9(3):e90233. https://doi.org/10.1371/journal.pone.0090233.

126. Wolak T, Aliev E, Rogachev B, et al. Renal safety and angiotensin II blockade medications in patients undergoing non-emergent coronary angiography: A randomized controlled study. Article. Isr Med Assoc J 2013;15(11):682–7.

127. Bainey KR, Rahim S, Etherington K, et al. Effects of withdrawing vs continuing renin-angiotensin blockers on incidence of acute kidney injury in patients with renal insufficiency undergoing cardiac catheterization: Results from the Angiotensin Converting Enzyme Inhibitor/Angiotensin Receptor Blocker and Contrast Induced Nephropathy in Patients Receiving Cardiac Catheterization (CAPTAIN) trial. Am Heart J 2015;170(1):110–6.

128. Rosenstock JL, Bruno R, Kim JK, et al. The effect of withdrawal of ACE inhibitors or angiotensin receptor blockers prior to coronary angiography on the incidence of contrast-induced nephropathy. Int Urol Nephrol 2008;40(3):749–55.

129. Desai M, Ram R, Prayaga A, et al. Cholesterol crystal embolization (CCE): Improvement of renal function with high-dose corticosteroid treatment. Saudi J Kidney Dis Transpl 2011;22(2):327–30.

130. Belenfant X, Meyrier A, Jacquot C. Supportive treatment improves survival in multivisceral cholesterol crystal embolism. Am J Kidney Dis 1999;33(5):840–50.

131. Dahlberg PJ, Frecentese DF, Cogbill TH. Cholesterol embolism: experience with 22 histologically proven cases. Surgery. Jun 1989;105(6):737–46.

132. Woolfson RG, Lachmann H. Improvement in renal cholesterol emboli syndrome after simvastatin. Lancet 1998;351(9112):1331–2.

133. Abela GS, Vedre A, Janoudi A, et al. Effect of statins on cholesterol crystallization and atherosclerotic plaque stabilization. Am J Cardiol 2011;107(12):1710–7.

134. Scolari F, Ravani P, Pola A, et al. Predictors of renal and patient outcomes in atheroembolic renal disease: a prospective study. J Am Soc Nephrol 2003;14(6):1584–90.

135. Keen RR, McCarthy WJ, Shireman PK, et al. Surgical management of atheroembolization. J Vasc Surg 1995;21(5):773–80 [discussion: 780-1].

Renalism: Avoiding Procedure, More Harm than Good?

Radha K. Adusumilli, MD[a], Steven Coca, DO, MS[b],*

KEYWORDS

- Chronic kidney disease • Contrast-associated nephropathy • Acute kidney injury • Renalism

KEY POINTS

- "Renalism," a concept coined by Chertow and colleagues, is an alteration in practice because of an aversion to the risk of acute kidney injury (AKI) or progression of chronic kidney disease (CKD).
- AKI is associated with worse outcomes such as CKD progression, end-stage renal disease, and cardiovascular morbidity and mortality. However, it is prudent to understand and differentiate, if AKI is the mediator or the markers of underlying comorbidity burden responsible for these poor outcomes.
- Understand the limitations of statistical adjustments for the confounding factors.
- Current definitions are too sensitive to identify AKI and cannot differentiate between transient hemodynamics alterations and tubular injury.
- A careful assessment of risks and benefits rather a blanket "do not harm" policy is needed to avoid renalism and offer optimal intervention opportunities to the CKD patients.

INTRODUCTION

"Renalism," a concept coined by Chertow and colleagues[1], is an alteration in practice because of an aversion to the risk of radiocontrast-associated nephrotoxicity. In the current era, it can pertain to withholding or delaying any intervention, be it percutaneous coronary angiography, coronary artery bypass surgery, underutilization or holding diuretics in cardio-renal syndrome, underutilization of renin–angiotensin–aldosterone inhibitors and sodium glucose cotransporter 2 inhibitors (SGLT2is), in an attempt to avoid an acute kidney injury (AKI).

The deep irony of renalism is that the risk–treatment paradox is usually in direct contradistinction to what should be done for the patient and in some ways can be viewed as a system-wide health care disparity for a vulnerable group

of patients with a significant burden of disease. With a prevailing perception of "do no harm," clinicians self-perpetuate the bias and unknowingly subvert optimal care for patients as a tradeoff for short-term gain of avoidance of largely transient decreases in serum creatinine. In this article, the authors discuss the phenomenon "renalism," the reasons behind it, the misconceptions that persist, and a path forward to break the bias and improve care for people with chronic kidney disease (CKD).

ORIGINS OF RENALISM

Chertow and colleagues[1] coined the term "renalism" based on their seminal analysis demonstrating that high-risk patients with CKD including the elderly received conservative treatment options despite the potential of coronary angiograph to have a meaningful impact

[a] UTHSCSA, San Antonio, TX, USA; [b] Icahn School of Medicine at Mount Sinai, One Gustave L. Levy Place, Box 1243, New York, NY 10029, USA
* Corresponding author.
E-mail address: steven.coca@mssm.edu
Twitter: @scoca1 (S.C.)

Intervent Cardiol Clin 12 (2023) 573–578
https://doi.org/10.1016/j.iccl.2023.06.005

on the patients' morbidity and mortality. In their retrospective analysis of final cohort of 57,284 patients, they used propensity scores to stratify patients with and without CKD on their likelihood of undergoing coronary angiography during hospitalization. The propensity score incorporated patient and hospital characteristics including demographics parameters, comorbidities, physiologic derangements in the blood work and other diagnostics, hospital characteristics of the initial admitting hospital, and interaction of selected factors in the model. In addition, among 92 clinical indications related to angiography during the initial hospitalization, the appropriateness score was determined using a combination of the following factors: duration of symptom onset (<6 hour, 6 to 12 hour, or >12 hour); age (<75 or ≥75 year); eligibility for and receipt of thrombolytic therapy; and the presence of complications such as persistent or recurrent chest pain, stress-induced ischemia, and pulmonary edema. The appropriateness scores ranged from 1 (extremely inappropriate) to 5 (uncertain) to 9 (extremely appropriate). An indication was categorized as necessary (angiography is the best option available to the patient), appropriate but not necessary (the benefits of performing angiography exceed the risks), uncertain (the benefits and risks are approximately equal), or inappropriate (the risks outweigh the benefits). In this analysis, they considered cases that were either necessary or appropriate anytime during their admission (deemed "appropriate") as having an indication for angiography to conservatively bias the analysis.[1] Overall, authors found that the older patients, women, and black individuals were less likely to undergo coronary angiography than the younger patients, men, and white individuals, respectively. In analyses comparing CKD versus non-CKD group, the rates of intervention were 25.2% and 46.8%, respectively (P < 0.0001). CKD patients with comorbidities such as congestive heart failure, stroke, low ejection fraction, and shock in hospital were less likely to get a coronary angiography. Adjusting for predictors of angiography, the odds ratio (OR) for angiography for CKD patients was 0.47 (95% confidence interval [CI], 0.40 to 0.52). Most importantly, after adjusting for other factors associated with 1-year mortality, coronary angiography was associated with a significant reduction in the risk of death (adjusted OR, 0.54; 95% CI, 0.49 to 0.60) in CKD patients. The incidence of contrast-associated AKI (CA-AKI) was not assessed.[1]

THE CAUSE OF RENALISM

Multiple studies over the last 2 decades have shown that AKI, even if mild and transient, is associated with a higher risk of poor outcomes including new onset or progressive CKD, cardiovascular events, and mortality.[2–7] In a retrospective study by Matthew and colleagues of 14,782 adults who received coronary angiography in the province of Alberta, Canada, between 2004 and 2006, 9.6% patients sustained AKI based on the AKI network criteria. In the Cox regression analysis, the adjusted risk of death, end-stage renal disease, cardiovascular, and renal hospitalizations increased with increasing severity of AKI compared with no AKI.[2] In another prospective multicenter cohort study of acute myocardial infarction patients who survived hospitalization, a worsening renal function was independently associated with a higher risk of death (hazard ratio [HR] 1.64, 95% CI 1.23 to 2.19) after adjustment of potential risk factors.[3]

Over the years, the thresholds to define AKI have moved to very sensitive definitions requiring just a 0.3 mg/dL increase in serum creatinine from the baseline to meet the criteria for AKI (stage I), as implemented in the latest and widely used KDIGO guidelines as well. AKI network criteria used in the study by Matthew and colleagues where 77% of AKI cases were stage I AKI.[2,8,9] Although these criteria have led to the widespread awareness and recognition of AKI by scientists and clinicians, there have been unintended adverse consequences of wide implementation of such sensitive definitions. An omission of necessary interventions which can be associated with mild increase in creatinine is one such consequence.

WHY FEAR ACUTE KIDNEY INJURY?

As aforementioned, AKI is associated with worse clinical outcomes despite adjustment for clinical covariates suggesting that AKI is an independent risk factor for the worse outcomes. It is important to note that the most AKI occurs spontaneously in the setting of acute illnesses such as heart failure exacerbation, sepsis, hemodynamics instability, and more frequently with baseline CKD. These settings are where most of the interventions (diagnostic and therapeutic) are required. For instance, in the study by Matthew and colleagues of those that developed stage 2 or 3 AKI, 42% had diabetes compared with 25% in those that did not develop AKI. Other comorbidities such as heart failure, cerebrovascular disease, peripheral vascular disease, chronic pulmonary disease were also higher at baseline in those with versus without AKI.[2] Thus, one can argue that AKI largely is a marker of the underlying comorbidity burden rather the consequence of the interventions. In the single-arm observational analyses, the mere adjustment of these illnesses as confounding covariates is not enough. It is well-known that residual confounding is always present due to known and unknown confounders as well as lack of granularity in some recognized potential covariates (eg, one can adjust for hypotension as a 1/0 variable or can use the systolic blood pressure, diastolic BP, mean arterial pressure, minimum BP, duration of hypotension).

Despite the known limitations of the AKI literature, the significance of AKI has permeated clinical practice and, in cases, where AKI can be preventable, has led to changes in care models to avoid AKI. Most of the clinical settings where AKI can be avoided are before a known procedure or imaging study (eg, angiography, CT with contrast) due to the extensive literature on CA-AKI. Indeed, countless preventative strategies have been suggested and investigated to mitigate CA-AKI (many of which have been later shown to have little or no effect on future outcomes).

CAN PREVENTING ACUTE KIDNEY INJURY IMPROVE WORSE OUTCOMES?

Most of the trials evaluating strategies to prevent CA-AKI examined short-term serum creatinine-based outcomes, not the hard clinical outcomes. With this in mind, the PRESERVE (Prevention of Serious Adverse Outcomes Following Angiography) trial was conducted to assess the effects of n-acetylcysteine (NAC) or intravenous (IV) bicarbonate or the combination compared with IV normal saline, in a 2 × 2 factorial design, on composite endpoint of death, need for dialysis, or persistent impairment in kidney function at 90 days. CA-AKI, defined as an increase in the serum creatinine of $\geq$0.5 mg/dL and/or $\geq$25% on the days 3 to 5 assessment compared with the pre-angiography level, was a secondary endpoint.[10] This multicenter international trial enrolled 5117 high-risk patients with estimated glomerular filtration rate (eGFR) of 15 to 44.9 mL/min/1.73 m^2 or an eGFR of 45 to 59.9 mL/min/1.73 m^2 with diabetes mellitus, who were scheduled to undergo either nonemergent coronary or noncoronary angiography. There was no effect of NAC, bicarbonate, or the combination on any of the sustained primary outcomes, nor was there a difference in the incidence of CA-AKI between the arms. Overall, the

incidence of AKI was 9.7%, but the incidence of sustained kidney injury-related outcomes was only 4.3%: 12.4% in those with AKI and 3.5% in those without AKI. Thus, patients with AKI had $\approx$ 4-fold increased risk of developing sustained kidney events even after adjusting for multiple confounders.[10] However, this long-awaited trial was incapable of assessing the association between AKI (specifically CA-AKI) and outcomes as a potential causal relationship due to the lack of protective effect of the intervention. Later, in a formal mediation analysis of the same data, it was interpreted that CA-AKI did not mediate the association of pre-angiography eGFR with 90-day death, need for dialysis or persistent kidney impairment.[11]

Similar findings were observed in the AMAastricht Contrast-Induced Nephropathy Guideline trial, which was a single-center, randomized controlled trial in patients with eGFR 30–59 mL/min/1.73 m^2, combined with risk factors, undergoing elective procedures requiring IV or intra-arterial iodinated contrast material. It compared prophylactic hydration with no hydration and evaluated dialysis, mortality, and change in renal function at 35 days as well as at 1 year.[12,13] The CA-AKI occurred in 2.65% of 603 total participants with no difference in hydration versus no hydration group. No hemodialysis or death occurred within 35 days. The HR was 1.118 (no prophylaxis vs prophylaxis) for 1-year risk of death (95% CI 0.70 to 1.80, $P = 0.6449$) and there was no difference in the rate of dialysis also. We conducted a meta-analysis of 14 RCTs that used interventions that influenced the incidence of AKI (not exclusive to CA-AKI) or acute changes in serum creatinine to quantify the relationship between positive or negative short-term effects of interventions on change in serum creatinine level and more meaningful clinical outcomes. We were unable to detect differences in the outcomes of CKD or mortality on follow-up, despite large effect sizes of a $\geq$50% increase or 40% decrease in the AKI end point.[14]

IS CONTRAST-ASSOCIATED-ACUTE KIDNEY INJURY REPRESENTATIVE OF TRUE KIDNEY INJURY?

The rise in serum creatinine after exposure to contrast does not always mean injury to the nephron. Indeed, in a subset of the PRESERVE trial, plasma and urinary biomarkers of kidney injury (kidney injury molecule-1, neutrophil gelatinase-associated lipocalin, IL-18) and repair (monocyte chemoattractant protein-1, uromodulin, YKL-40) proteins were measured at baseline and 2 to 4 hours post-angiography.[15] The investigators assessed the associations between absolute changes and relative ratios of biomarkers with CA-AKI and 90-day major adverse kidney events (MAKEs) and death. The participants ($n = 922$) were predominately men (97%) with diabetes (82%). No post-angiography urine biomarkers were associated with CA-AKI. Moreover, the absolute change and relative ratios of plasma and urine biomarkers were modest and comparable between patients with and without CA-AKI. In an additional study using the same urine and blood samples, highly sensitive kidney cell cycle arrest and cardiac biomarkers were assessed.[16] There were no differences in post-angiography urinary tissue inhibitor of matrix metalloproteinase-2 and insulin growth factor binding protein-7, plasma brain natriuretic peptide, serum troponin, and high-sensitive C-reactive protein concentrations among patients with and without CA-AKI and MAKEs. These findings suggested that there is no evidence of intrinsic kidney injury in CA-AKI. In these analyses, the magnitudes of the absolute changes of the six plasma and urine biomarkers in this study were much smaller when compared with cohorts of cardiac surgery recipients and marathon runners.[17,18]

Summarizing the above observations: CA-AKI occurred without any benefit of the interventions on sustained outcomes, and AKI episodes associated with worse outcomes; however, the diagnosis of AKI was mostly based on change in creatinine without substantial absolute changes in the biomarkers of kidney injury, and in formal mediation analysis, AKI did not mediate the worse outcomes. The potential explanation for these observations is that the majority of increases in serum creatinine that defined CA-AKI were due to hemodynamic fluctuations leading to altered renal and glomerular blood flow rather than injury which probably reflects the underlying comorbidities burden compromising the renal reserve.[19] Therefore, the interventions might or not prevent the change in creatinine but could not impact the sustained kidney outcomes; however, patients had long-term worse outcomes such as death, cardiovascular (CV) disease as a result of underlying comorbidities introducing residual confounding which statistical analyses could not adjust for.

THE CONSEQUENCES OF RENALISM

What are the true consequences of renalism? Weisbord and colleagues[20] conducted a retrospective analysis of US Veterans hospitalized at Veterans Affairs (VA) Medical Centers from January 2013 to December 2017 and had a discharge diagnosis of acute coronary syndrome (ACS). They used multivariable logistic regression to investigate the association of CKD with the use of invasive care (coronary angiography, with or without revascularization; coronary artery bypass graft surgery; or both) deemed clinically indicated based on Global Registry of Acute Coronary Events 2.0 risk scores that predicted 6-month all-cause mortality $\geq 5\%$. Using propensity scoring and inverse probability weighting, they also examined the association of nonuse of clinically indicated invasive care with 6-month all-cause mortality, after adjusting for age, sex, race, VA facility, Cath laboratory volume, blood pressures, pulse, diuretic use, change in troponin, ST deviation, and comorbidities in Gagne comorbidity score. Among 34,430 patients with a clinical indication for invasive care, those with CKD were less likely than those without CKD to receive clinically indicated care (adjusted OR 0.68; 95% CI, 0.65 to 0.72). Among patients with CKD, nonuse of invasive care was associated with higher risk of 6-month all-cause mortality (absolute risk, 21.5% vs 15.5%; absolute risk difference 6.0%; adjusted risk ratio [RR], 1.39; 95% CI, 1.29 to 1.49). Their findings were consistent across multiple sensitivity analyses. They also observed more renalism with more advanced CKD. The adjusted OR (95% CI) for clinically indicated invasive care was 0.9 (0.85–0.96), 0.61 (0.57–0.65), and 0.40 (0.32–0.39) for CKD 3a, CKD 3b, and CKD 4, respectively. It was noted that there was no increased risk of AKI in those with invasive care versus non-invasive care (adjusted OR 1.03, 95% CI 0.96–1.10).[20] The striking risk–treatment paradox by CKD and severity of CKD observed in the VA data despite robust data that indicate that invasive care for ACS in those with CKD is associated with a markedly reduced the risk of death. A meta-analysis of nearly 150,000 patients with ACS from large observational studies as well as five randomized controlled trials demonstrated nearly 50% lower mortality with early invasive care compared with early noninvasive treatment among observational studies (RR = 0.53, 95% CI, 0.45 to 0.62).[21]

The main driver of renalism, after the review of the data above, likely relates to the widespread misconception that AKI post-angiography is a mediator of mortality rather than a marker of severity of illness. As analogized by Dr Weisbord, the renalism bias is akin to the treatment of atrial fibrillation. Choudhry and colleagues[22] observed that physicians who had a patient with a major bleed and had treated other patients with atrial fibrillation, had a 21% decrease in the prescription of anticoagulation over next 3 months. On the contrary, the physicians who cared for patients who developed stroke while not on anticoagulation were not more likely to prescribe anticoagulation in the subsequent period. The conclusion is that acts of commission are perceived as more harmful than acts of omission, meaning doing no harm by not intervening is perceived to be less harmful than placing a patient at risk of a complication. The same mindset among clinicians is likely operative for patients with CKD needing invasive procedures.

SUMMARY

It is clear that the fear of AKI and rise in creatinine should not be a reason to withhold otherwise clinically indicated management in patients with CKD. On the contrary, because cardiovascular disease is the leading cause of morbidity and mortality in patients with CKD, with clear evidence that withholding of invasive procedures leads to worse outcomes in patients with CKD, efforts to proceed with these procedures should be maximized. Indeed, the risk of AKI in the modern era is minimal at best, is largely hemodynamic without true tubule injury, is largely transient, and the benefits at a population level for CKD far outweigh the risks. It needs to be pointed out that there is a certain selected patient population at high risk for CA-AKI and potential for need for renal replacement therapy. The use of contemporary validated risk prediction calculators such as Mehran score[23] to determine those patients are advised followed by selection of the best approach after careful discussion between the treating clinicians and the patient. However, for many patients with CKD, the mindset of renalism by clinicians must be markedly changed to achieve better outcomes for this venerable patient population.

CLINICS CARE POINTS

- Avoidance of the potential for AKI by withholding of a cardiovascular procedure may provide harm to the patient.
- The risks associated with AKI are less than that of unmitigated cardiovascular disease.
- Risk scores to calculate the risk for contrast-associated AKI may be helpful in clinical practice.

DISCLOSURE

S. Coca reports the following: Employer: Icahn School of Medicine at Mount Sinai; Mount Sinai owns part of Renalytix; Consultancy: Renalytix, Takeda, Nuwellis, Vifor, Bayer, Boehringer-Ingelheim, Reprieve Cardiovascular, Axon, 3ive; Ownership Interest: Renalytix, pulseData; Patents or Royalties: Renalytix; and Other Interests or Relationships: Associate Editor for Kidney360, Editorial Boards of JASN, CJASN, Kidney International.

REFERENCES

1. Chertow GM, Normand SL, McNeil BJ. "Renalism": inappropriately low rates of coronary angiography in elderly individuals with renal insufficiency. J Am Soc Nephrol 2004;15(9):2462–8.
2. James MT, Ghali WA, Knudtson ML, et al. Hemmelgarn and for the alberta provincial project for outcome assessment in coronary heart disease (APPROACH) Investigators: associations between acute kidney injury and cardiovascular and renal outcomes after coronary angiography. Circulation 2011;123:409–16.
3. Amin AP, Spertus JA, Reid KJ, et al. The prognostic importance of worsening renal function during an acute myocardial infarction on long-term mortality. Am Heart J 2010;160(6):1065–71. ISSN 0002-8703.
4. Spertus JA, Peterson E, Rumsfeld JS, et al. The prospective registry evaluating myocardial infarction: events and recovery (PREMIER)—evaluating the impact of myocardial infarction on patient outcomes. Am Heart J 2006;151:589–97.
5. Forman DE, et al. Incidence, predictors at admission, and impact of worsening renal function among patients hospitalized with heart failure. J Am Coll Cardiol 2004;43(1):61–7.
6. Smith GL, Vaccarino V, Kosiborod M, et al. Worsening renal function: what is a clinically meaningful change in creatinine during hospitalization with heart failure? J Card Fail 2003;9(1):13–25.
7. Ferrer-Hita JJ, Dominguez-Rodriguez A, Garcia-Gonzalez MJ, et al. Renal dysfunction is an independent predictor of in-hospital mortality in patients with ST-segment elevation myocardial infarction treated with primary angioplasty. Int J Cardiol 2007;118(2):243–5.
8. Mehta RL, Kellum JA, Shah SV, et al. Acute kidney injury network: report of an initiative to improve outcomes in acute kidney injury. Crit Care 2007; 11(2):R31.
9. KDIGO clinical practice guideline for the management of blood pressure in chronic kidney disease. Kidney Int 2012;2(5):85.
10. Weisbord SD, Gallagher M, Jneid H, et al. for the PRESERVE trial group outcomes after angiography

with sodium bicarbonate and acetylcysteine. N Engl J Med 2018;378:603–14.

11. Weisbord SD, Palevsky PM, Kaufman JS, et al. Contrast-associated acute kidney injury and serious adverse outcomes following angiography. J Am Coll Cardiol 2020;75(11):1311–20. ISSN 0735-1097.

12. Nijssen EC, Rennenberg RJ, Nelemans PJ, et al. Prophylactic hydration to protect renal function from intravascular iodinated contrast material in patients at high risk of contrast-induced nephropathy (AMACING): a prospective, randomised, phase 3, controlled, open-label, non-inferiority trial. Lancet 2017;389(10076):1312–22.

13. Nijssen EC, Nelemans PJ, Rennenberg RJ, et al. Prophylactic intravenous hydration to protect renal function from intravascular iodinated contrast material (AMACING): long-term results of a prospective, randomised, controlled trial. EClinicalMedicine 2018;4-5:109–16.

14. Coca SG, Zabetian A, Ferket BS, et al. Evaluation of short-term changes in serum creatinine level as a meaningful end point in randomized clinical trials. J Am Soc Nephrol 2016;27(8):2529–42.

15. Liu C, Mor MK, Palevsky PM, et al. Postangiography increases in serum creatinine and biomarkers of injury and repair. CJASN 2020;15(9):1240–50.

16. Murugan R, Boudreaux-Kelly MY, Kellum JA, et al. Biomarker effectiveness analysis in contrast nephropathy (BEACON) study investigators kidney cell cycle arrest and cardiac biomarkers and acute kidney injury following angiography: the prevention of serious adverse events following angiography (PRESERVE) study. Kidney Med 2022;5(3):100592.

17. Parikh CR, Thiessen-Philbrook H, Garg AX, et al, TRIBE-AKI Consortium. Performance of kidney injury molecule-1 and liver fatty acid-binding protein and combined biomarkers of AKI after cardiac surgery. Clin J Am Soc Nephrol 2013;8:1079–88.

18. Mansour SG, Verma G, Pata RW, et al. Kidney injury and repair biomarkers in marathon runners. Am J Kidney Dis 2017;70:252–61. published correction appears in AmJ KidneyDis 70: 452, 2017.

19. Palsson R, Waikar SS. Renal functional reserve revisited. Adv Chron Kidney Dis 2018;25(3):e1–8.

20. Weisbord SD, Mor MK, Hochheiser H, et al. Utilization and outcomes of clinically indicated invasive cardiac care in veterans with acute coronary syndrome and chronic kidney disease. J Am Soc Nephrol 2023;34(4):694–705.

21. Shaw C, Nitsch D, Lee J, et al. Impact of an early invasive strategy versus conservative strategy for unstable angina and non-ST elevation acute coronary syndrome in patients with chronic kidney disease: a systematic review. PLoS One 2016;11(5):e0153478.

22. Choudhry NK, Anderson GM, Laupacis A, et al. Impact of adverse events on prescribing warfarin in patients with atrial fibrillation: matched pair analysis. BMJ 2006;332:141.

23. Mehran R, Owen R, Chiarito M, et al. A contemporary simple risk score for prediction of contrast-associated acute kidney injury after percutaneous coronary intervention: derivation and validation from an observational registry. Lancet 2021;398(10315):1974–83.

Moving?

Make sure your subscription moves with you!

To notify us of your new address, find your **Clinics Account Number** (located on your mailing label above your name), and contact customer service at:

Email: journalscustomerservice-usa@elsevier.com

800-654-2452 (subscribers in the U.S. & Canada)
314-447-8871 (subscribers outside of the U.S. & Canada)

Fax number: 314-447-8029

Elsevier Health Sciences Division
Subscription Customer Service
3251 Riverport Lane
Maryland Heights, MO 63043

*To ensure uninterrupted delivery of your subscription, please notify us at least 4 weeks in advance of move.

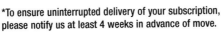

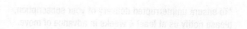

Printed and bound by CPI Group (UK) Ltd, Croydon, CR0 4YY

03/10/2024

01040365-0010